Elizabeth Connor, MLS, AHIP

Internet Guide to Anti-Aging and Longevity

Pre-publication
REVIEW . . .

"In the chaotic morass of information that is the Internet, the *Internet Guide to Anti-Aging and Longevity* is a welcome guidebook for a topic that is increasingly on everyone's mind. The work covers not only the expected and traditional subjects that concern an aging population but also some that are innovative, yet still important. Web sites that address the issues of bone and joint disorders, hair and hearing loss, and incontinence are well covered as are pet ownership, relationship issues, and 'fringe' areas such as cryogenics and herbal medicine.

This guide is well organized and includes a useful glossary for those not as learned in the vocabulary of the Internet and Web sites. I found the brief introduction to the Internet and World Wide Web helpful. It was short enough not to bore knowledgeable audiences, and had enough meat to empower those new to this arena.

This is a useful guide to online health information for the educated consumer. It is appropriate for any size library collection and should find its place in almost anyone's personal library."

Stephen L. Clancy, MLS, AHIP
*Research Librarian for Medicine
and Acting Medicine Education Coordinator,
Reference Department, Science Library,
University of California, Irvine*

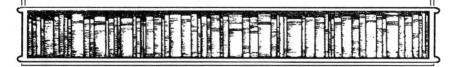

Internet Guide to Anti-Aging and Longevity

THE HAWORTH INFORMATION PRESS®
Haworth Internet Medical Guides
M. Sandra Wood, MLS
Editor

The Guide to Complementary and Alternative Medicine on the Internet by Lillian R. Brazin

Internet Guide to Travel Health by Elizabeth Connor

Internet Guide to Food Safety and Security by Elizabeth Connor

Internet Guide to Cosmetic Surgery for Women by M. Sandra Wood

Internet Guide to Anti-Aging and Longevity by Elizabeth Connor

Internet Guide to Cosmetic Surgery for Men by M. Sandra Wood

Internet Guide to Anti-Aging and Longevity

Elizabeth Connor, MLS, AHIP

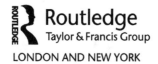

Routledge
Taylor & Francis Group

LONDON AND NEW YORK

First published 2006 by The Haworth Press, Inc.

2 Park Square, Milton Park, Abingdon, Oxfordshire OX14 4RN
605 Third Avenue, New York, NY 10017

Routledge is an imprint of the Taylor & Francis Group, an informa business

First issued in hardback 2020

Cover design by Marylouise E. Doyle.

Library of Congress Cataloging-in-Publication Data

Connor, Elizabeth, MLS.
    Internet guide to anti-aging and longevity / Elizabeth Connor.
       p. cm.
    Includes bibliographical references and index.
    ISBN-13: 978-0-7890-2860-0 (hc. : alk. paper)
    ISBN-10: 0-7890-2860-3 (hc. : alk. paper)
    ISBN-13: 978-0-7890-2861-7 (pbk. : alk. paper)
    ISBN-10: 0-7890-2861-1 (pbk. : alk. paper)
    1. Aging—Prevention—Computer network resources—Directories. 2. Longevity—Computer network resources—Directories. 3. Health—Computer network resources—Directories. 4. Internet addresses—Directories. 5. Web sites—Directories. I. Title.
    [DNLM: 1. Aging—Resource Guides. 2. Health Education—Aged—Resource Guides. 3. Health Promotion—Aged—Resource Guides. 4. Internet—Resource Guides. 5. Longevity—Resource Guides. WT 39 C753i 2006]

RA776.75.C6613 2006
025.06'132—dc22

                                              2005016684

ISBN 13: 978-0-7890-2860-0 (hbk)

In memory of Peter Jas. Houle (1954-2004)
whose years will never end

ABOUT THE AUTHOR

Elizabeth Connor, MLS, AHIP, is Assistant Professor of Library Science and Science Liaison at the Daniel Library of the Citadel, Charleston, South Carolina, and is a distinguished member of the Academy of Health Information Professionals. Ms. Connor spent several years in leadership positions at major teaching hospitals and academic medical centers in Maryland, Connecticut, South Carolina, Saudi Arabia, and the Commonwealth of Dominica. She is the author of several peer-reviewed articles about medical informatics, electronic resources, search engines, and chat reference, and has written more than sixty book reviews for *Library Journal, Against the Grain, Bulletin of the Medical Library Association, Journal of the Medical Library Association, Medical Reference Services Quarterly, Doody's Reviews,* and *The Post & Courier.* Ms. Connor manages the book review process for *Medical References Services Quarterly* and is the co-editor of *Journal of Electronic Resources in Medical Libraries.* Ms. Connor is the author of the *Internet Guide to Travel Health, Internet Guide to Food Safety and Security, A Guide to Developing End User Education Programs in Medical Libraries,* and *Planning, Renovating, and Constructing Library Facilities in Hospitals, Academic Medical Centers, and Health Organizations,* all published by The Haworth Press.

CONTENTS

Preface

Health consumers and health professionals alike seek authoritative, reliable, and up-to-date information about habits, practices, and factors that promote long life and help fight the sometimes debilitating effects of aging. Controversies include hormone therapy, antioxidants, macrobiotic diets, food supplements, and the like. Some commercial enterprises and organizations promote drastic exercise regimens and unproven medical treatments such as cell transplantation to extend the quality of life beyond average life expectancy. Until quite recently, the term *aged* or *elderly* referred to persons sixty years of age and older. Now persons fifty years of age and older refer to themselves as middle-aged, the word *senior* is used to describe persons sixty-five and older, and many people expect to stay active and healthy throughout their lives.

This comprehensive compilation of annotated links serves as a handy, useful, and easy-to-consult guide for persons of all ages who are interested in staying healthy and vital during every stage of life. Many diseases and conditions associated with aging are included here but complex topics such as cancer, cardiovascular diseases, cosmetic surgery, movement disorders, accidents, and Alzheimer's disease are not covered in depth. A number of research areas hold implications for current and future understanding of aging processes, including studying centenarians, studying persons with progeria, a rare but serious condition that is characterized by extreme onset of aging in children, and comparing aging and longevity in twins. The predominant emphasis is on English-language information from North American sites, with some links from the United Kingdom, Australia, and some European countries.

Remember to consult a physician before embarking on new treatments, diets, or exercise regimens. May you thrive and prosper in this wonderful and ever-changing world. Enjoy a long, fruitful, and healthy life surrounded by people who love you.

We grow old more through indolence, than through age.

Christina, Queen of Sweden

Chapter 1

Introduction

Understanding the effects of aging and living a long and healthy life involve planning, preparation, and awareness of heredity, healthy lifestyles, unhealthy situations, and potential health risks. Researchers and health practitioners consider aging to be a natural and lifelong process that starts as soon as life itself begins, and believe that a combination of factors including genetics, environment, health care, and moderate lifestyle habits (diet, exercise, temperament) contribute to how long or well a person lives. U.S. government demographers predict that by the year 2025, more than 327,000 Americans will be 100 years of age or older.[1] Over time, the average life expectancy at birth has increased by more than seven years, from 70.8 years in 1970 to 77.2 years in 2001.[2]

Recent research studies have noted a correlation between eating what is known as a Mediterranean diet and habits including walking, moderate use of alcohol, and nonsmoking with the prevention of dementia in the elderly.[3] Mediterranean diet is a vague term that refers to the consumption of small amounts of animal proteins and dairy products supplemented by large amounts of fresh fruits, vegetables, whole grains, and olive oil. The Seven Countries Study conducted by Ancel Keys looked at the relationship among diet, cholesterol levels, and heart disease.[4] Keys was a physiologist who studied the physiology of food deprivation and starvation, eating habits in Mediterranean countries, physiological effects of altitude, and related subjects.

Pockets of longevity, meaning relatively large numbers of persons living well into their eighties, nineties, and beyond, have been noted in various geographic regions such as island nations and regions in Dominica, Japan, and Sicily and in isolated and mountainous regions such as Azerbaijan, northern Italy, and Tibet. Some suggest that isolation caused by bodies of water and mountainous terrain may reduce the risk of disease. Much can be learned from reading about the lifestyles of persons with extraordinarily long life spans.[5]

Curious and discerning individuals can use the Internet to find updated and authoritative information on a variety of topics, including consumer health. The Internet has the potential to improve health knowledge, and to increase awareness of health risks. The Pew Internet & American Life Project reports that "fifty-two million American adults, or 55 percent of those with Internet access, have used the Web to get health or medical information."[6]

ANATOMY OF A WEB SITE ADDRESS

Hypertext transfer protocol (http) is the set of standards that is used to represent content on the World Wide Web. Although many Web browsers no longer require the http:// prefix when entering site addresses, other prefixes are understood by browser software to connect to other types of Internet resources. For example, the telnet:// prefix is used to establish a telnet connection, which allows remote users to log-in to resources such as electronic catalogs of library holdings. The ftp:// prefix signifies file transfer protocol that is used to transmit files from one computer to another. Each Web site address is comprised of distinct and meaningful parts that describe the host computer, directory, and file name:

<protocol://host.domain.suffix.suffix/directory>

For example, in the address <http://www.hhp.ufl.edu/keepingfit>, hhp (Health and Human Performance) is the host name, ufl (University of Florida) is the domain, edu indicates an educational institution, and keepingfit is the directory. In the address for MedlinePlus's information about medical news, <http://www.nlm.nih.gov/medlineplus/newsbydate.html>, the domain is the National Library of Medicine (NLM) at the National Institutes of Health (NIH), a group of government agencies (.gov), the directory is MedlinePlus, and the file name is newsbydate.

Many Web users are familiar with the use of file extensions such as .htm, .html, and .pdf at the end of site addresses. Hypertext markup language (html) is used to create and display Web content, as indicated by .htm or .html at the end of file names, but use of these suffixes is seen less frequently because of changes in site design. Web designers that use "server-side includes" (SSI) use .shtml instead of .htm or .html. Documents in Adobe's portable document format use the .pdf extension. Dynamic files created with ColdFusion software may have .cfm at the end.

Although .php originally meant personal home page, it now means hypertext preprocessor, signifying the use of server-side scripting language. Sites that use Java scripting software may show .jsp (Java server pages) as part of the file name. If a site uses Microsoft scripting software instead of Java, the file suffix is .asp (active server pages).

The ease with which Web sites are designed and content can be uploaded has resulted in many temporary, redesigned, or outdated sites. Dead links result when a site changes file names, alters the site navigation, or stops publishing. If a particular site address no longer functions, delete the /directory, /filename.htm, or /filename.html part of the address, and use the host.domain.suffix parts. After the site loads, use the site's search function (if one exists) to find the specific document or section needed. If this approach does not work, try the "wayback machine" <http://www.archive.org/web/web.php>, which provides a simple search interface for searching billions of archived Web pages dating back to 1996.

Web site addresses can include organizational or geographic suffixes that are meaningful. Table 1.1 lists common address suffixes and their meanings. Commercial Web sites or sites with a .com suffix at the end of the address can include useful scientific content. Reputable educational institutions such as the Mayo Clinic and Johns Hopkins University, for example, maintain authoritative consumer health information on .com sites with content that is separate from their .edu sites. Some excellent consumer health sites sell brochures and other products, but the sites featured in this guide provide freely available information, including some sites that require completion of a registration process to personalize future site interactions, or association membership for full access to all content on the site.

TABLE 1.1. Site Type and Geographic Suffixes

Site type suffix	Geographic suffix
.com—Commercial sites	
.co.uk—Commercial sites in the United Kingdom	.au—Australia
.edu—Educational sites	.ca—Canada
.gov—Government sites	.ch—Switzerland
.mil—Military sites	.ie—Ireland
.net—Commercial sites that provide network services	.nz—New Zealand
.org—Organization or association sites	.uk—United Kingdom

EVALUATING WEB CONTENT

Consumers of health information should be careful about medical information or advice obtained through the Internet. The currency, accuracy, and source of health-related information are very important factors to consider. Laypersons should be as skeptical and particular as health professionals when distinguishing between anecdotal information and content derived from authoritative and peer-reviewed sources.

Health on the Net (HON) Foundation <http://www.hon.ch/> is an organization based in Switzerland that developed MedHunt, an English/French medical search engine, and a set of standards for evaluating sites with medical content (see Figure 1.1). The HON Code of Conduct rates Web sites according to whether a particular site with medical content provides the following:

- Explanation of qualifications for dispensing advice or developing content
- Maintenance of confidentiality when handling medical information
- Attribution of information derived from other sources
- Indication of when content was modified or revised
- Detailed contact information for content developers
- Identification of sources of funding or sponsorship
- Explanation of the site's use of advertisements or sale of products
- Differentiation between original content and promotional content

Health consumers may wish to pay close attention to the understandability of printed or online medical information. Medical jargon can be unfamiliar and confusing. Depending on individual levels of health knowledge and medical vocabulary, consumers should seek correspondingly

FIGURE 1.1. HON Code of Conduct (HONcode) Symbol for Medical and Health Web Sites
<http://www.hon/ch/>
Source: Health on the Net (HON) Foundation.
Used with permission.

simple or complex information. Readers can consult the glossary featured at the end of this book to better understand some of the terms used by persons involved in anti-aging, and longevity work and research.

SEARCH ENGINES/DIRECTORIES

Although Internet applications were developed as early as 1969 and allowed government agencies to communicate and share information, the part of the Internet known as the World Wide Web was not introduced until 1990. Gopher, the first Internet search tool, appeared in 1991, and earned its name due to its burrowing capabilities. The development of graphical browser tools (Mosaic, Netscape, Internet Explorer, Firefox) and sophisticated search engines/directories accelerated the growth, development, and acceptance of the World Wide Web. The widespread use of these freely available search tools has contributed to the evolution of Web searching into a daily activity, but often search queries yield thousands of marginally relevant results, with some dated or extinct links. Search engines have advantages and drawbacks, and it is worthwhile to learn the features of a few to serve a variety of needs.

A search engine delivers dynamically generated results based on the words typed into the search box. A search directory provides somewhat static groupings of categorized or preselected sites, and tends to be smaller in scope than a search engine. For subjects related to anti-aging and longevity, it may be more productive to focus on several sites with reliable, research-based health content (e.g., Food and Drug Administration, Centers for Disease Control and Prevention, National Library of Medicine's MedlinePlus, or World Health Organization) than to enter keywords into a search engine interface and spend hours sorting through links of dubious quality or authority.

Search engines/directories differ greatly in size and in how they are designed, compiled, updated, and organized. Search Engine Showdown <http://www.searchengineshowdown.com/> and Search Engine Watch <http://searchenginewatch.com/> are excellent sources of information about how specific search tools function and the relative size, advantages, and features of each. The following search engines/directories are useful for searching a variety of topics, and were used to locate the links included in this book:

- **Google** <http://www.google.com/>: Google is an excellent all-purpose resource for searching or browsing content including publicly accessible Web sites, news group messages, images, shopping price comparisons (Froogle), scholarly information (Google Scholar), and more. The subject categories in the Google Directory <http://directory.google.com/> can be browsed and searched. Features include the caching of old pages, linking to similar content, and narrowing results to specific universities, type of sites, type of file formats, and other variables.
- **Yahoo!** <http://www.yahoo.com/>: Yahoo!'s advantages as a search directory include compilation by humans, organization, speed, and ease of use. If Yahoo! exhausts its index, the search query is referred to its search engine. Features include image, news, local, and product searching.
- **Teoma** <http://www.teoma.com/>: Teoma is a crawler-based engine owned by Ask Jeeves <http://www.askjeeves.com/>. A crawler scours the World Wide Web, stores site addresses, and indexes the sites it finds. Useful features include the clustering of results retrieved from the same site and linking to more results.
- **Vivisimo** <http://www.vivisimo.com/>: Vivisimo is a metasearch engine with a useful clustering mechanism. Metasearch engines look at several search engines at once. A quick search on anti-aging yields a group of 250 sites clustered into different folders: Skin Care (63), Anti-Aging Products (44), Medicine (33), Human Growth Hormone (23), Research (15), Anti-Aging Therapies (13), Anti-Aging Center (9), and so forth.

Several search engines and directories focus on specific areas of interest such as government, medicine, or seniors. These specialized resources may be useful to research topics related to anti-aging and longevity:

- **FirstGov.gov** <http://www.firstgov.gov/>: FirstGov is the U.S. government's Web portal, an aggregated interface that can be used to search for content available on federal and state government sites. FirstGov for Science <http://www.science.gov/> is a portal subset that focuses on science, specifically authoritative information available from twelve U.S. government agencies, including the Departments of Agriculture, Commerce, Defense, Energy, Education, Health and Human Services, Interior; the Environmental Protection Agency;

NASA; the National Science Foundation; and the Government Printing Office. In addition to searching these agencies and their databases, it is possible to browse topic areas such as Agriculture & Food; Applied Science & Technology; Biology & Nature; Environment & Environmental Quality; and Health & Medicine, among others. FirstGov for Seniors <http://www.firstgov.gov/Topics/Seniors.shtml> focuses on consumer protection, education, jobs and volunteerism; federal and state agencies; health; retirement and money; taxes; and travel and leisure links of interest and value to older Americans, or Americans concerned with growing older (see Figure 1.2).

- **MedHunt** <http://www.hon.ch/medhunt/>: Health on the Net Foundation (HON) is known for its approval system for health-related sites. HON also maintains MedHunt as a medical search engine that annotates and ranks search results for more than 90,000 full-text documents. Search features include using logical operators (and, or, adjacent) and limiting results to geographic domains, news, images, HONcode sites, and conferences.
- **<http://searchedu.com> <http://searchmil.com> <http://searchgov. com>:** Despite the .com suffix on each of these site addresses, the interfaces retrieve results that are limited to education (.edu), military (.mil), and government (.gov) sites, respectively, making it easier to focus on authoritative content.
- **Scirus** <http://www.scirus.com/>: As of August 2005, Scirus "searches over 200 million science-specific Web pages." Scirus focuses on scientific, peer-reviewed journal content including e-prints, preprints (articles available before release of print publication), citations, and full-text literature (see Figure 1.3). Nonscientific sites are filtered out of the search results. Results can be restricted to specific years, journals, authors, and subjects within science, technology, and medicine.

DISCUSSION GROUPS, WEB FORUMS, AND BLOGS

The Internet has spawned online communities, Web forums, and Web logs (blogs) for persons with specialized interests. Researchers associated with the Pew Internet & American Life Project have estimated that as many as 27 percent of Americans who go online read blogs.[7] These resources allow people to share information through e-mail or Web-based

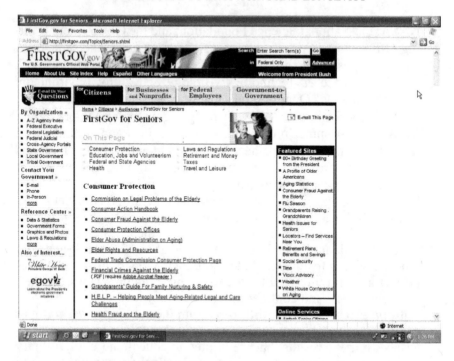

FIGURE 1.2. FirstGov for Seniors
<http://www.firstgov.gov/Topics/Seniors.shtml/>

interfaces. MetaFilter (MeFi) allows multiple persons to post content to the same Web-based log in a sequential, almost conversational way. These tools have revolutionized the dissemination of ideas and news, but some of the resulting content is inaccurate, unscientific, and unsubstantiated. Anecdotal information about health conditions and their treatments may be more harmful than helpful.

THE INVISIBLE WEB

The Invisible Web refers to content that is not easily retrieved or accessed through normal search engines because of the way some information is organized and how search engines find links. To tease out valuable content featured in deeper site layers or within some Web-based databases, try Search Adobe PDF Online <http://searchpdf.adobe.com>, InfoMine

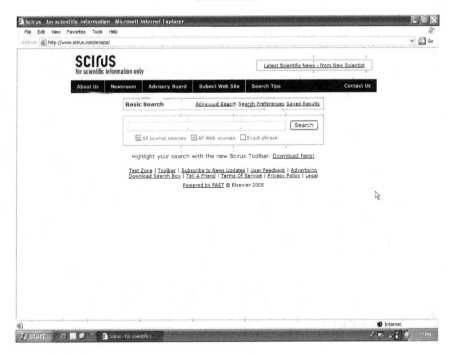

FIGURE 1.3. Scirus
<http://www.scirus.com/>
Reprinted with permission from Elsevier and Scirus.

<http://infomine.ucr.edu/>, ProFusion <http://www.profusion.com/>, or Spire Project Light <http://spireproject.com/spir.htm>.

STAYING HEALTHY AND WELL-INFORMED

To look and feel youthful, learn as much as you can about what makes you feel active and vital. Long life can be attributed to a combination of genetics, healthy living, moderate exercise, and good fortune. Consumers can improve their knowledge related to anti-aging and longevity by focusing on authoritative sources of information and avoiding unsubstantiated consumer health information.

Healthy People 2010 <http://www.healthypeople.gov/> is organized by the Office of Disease Prevention and Health Promotion and other U.S. federal agencies to encourage American citizens to take personal responsibility for their health by developing effective lifestyle habits, reducing health risks, and other strategies. Now more than at any other time in history, health knowledge, preventive measures, and treatments are available to improve and extend the quality of life for all.

UNSUBSTANTIATED INFORMATION

American society thrives on the dissemination of "urban legends," which are recent but largely untrue stories spread by word-of-mouth (and lately, by e-mail, online discussion groups, blogs, and Web sites) that can reach epic proportions. Health consumers should be aware of potential fraud and quackery when seeking information about anti-aging and longevity treatments and products. Fictitious examples related to anti-aging and longevity include sightings of Elvis Presley, keeping cells young with a mixture of Jack Daniel's whiskey and snuff juice, and transplantation of animal tissues to humans. Harmful and harmless elixirs, "snake oil," and potions have existed since the beginning of time; discerning consumers can consult a number of resources to understand and dispel unsubstantiated health claims.

Quackwatch SM <http://www.quackwatch.com/> is a corporation developed and maintained by Dr. Stephen Barrett, and its purpose is "to combat health-related frauds, myths, fads, and fallacies." The National Council Against Health Fraud (NCAHF) <http://www.ncahf.org/> is a useful resource for determining whether a particular health treatment is fraudulent or not and is also maintained by Dr. Barrett.

To help determine whether an anecdote is truth or folklore, consult Urban Legends Reference <http://www.snopes.com/>, Urban Legends and Folklore <http://urbanlegends.about.com/>, and Museum of Hoaxes <http://www.museumofhoaxes.com/> which collects data and reports on such stories.

SOURCES OF AUTHORITATIVE INFORMATION

Various government sites and universities that may focus on aspects of anti-aging and longevity research include the National Institute on Aging, the Institute of Medicine (IOM), U.S. Food and Drug Administration, U.S.

Administration on Aging, U.S. Social Security Administration, and resources developed by the National Library of Medicine.

The United States maintains two national libraries that provide services and resources which support scientific research and topics related to antiaging and longevity. The National Agricultural Library (NAL) <http://www.nal.usda.gov/> in Beltsville, Maryland, strives to improve life by providing access to agricultural information, most notably through its collections, services, and resources such as AGRICOLA, a bibliographic database that covers many aspects of agriculture, animal science, food and nutrition, water quality, and related subjects. The National Library of Medicine (NLM) <http://www.nlm.nih.gov/> in Bethesda, Maryland, is the largest biomedical library in the world and produces an array of bibliographic and full-text resources including MEDLINE and MedlinePlus.

Although this guide is intended to be as thorough as possible, use the sites marked with the ☑ symbol to save considerable time and effort when researching these subjects. Consult the glossary to learn the definitions of words that are unfamiliar. Scientific knowledge increases exponentially, and lifestyle, food habits, and health practices that were safe a few years ago can be dangerous today because of changes in economics, environment, and society.

NOTES

1. U.S. Census Bureau. *IDB Summary Demographic Data for United States.* Available online at <http://www.census.gov/>.

2. U.S. National Center for Health Statistics. Available online at <http://www.cdc.gov/nchs/fastats/lifexpec.htm>.

3. Knoops, K. T. B., de Groot, L. C. P. G. M., Kromhout, D., Perrin, A. E., Moreiras-Varela, O., Menotti, A., and Staveren, W. A., (2004). Mediterranean Diet, Lifestyle Factors, and 10-Year Mortality in Elderly European Men and Women: The HALE Project. *JAMA,* 292 (September 22/29): 1433-1439.

4. Keys, A., Aravanis, C., Blackburn, H., van Buchem, F. S. P., Buzina, R., and Djordjevic, B. S. (1967). Epidemiologic Studies Related to Coronary Heart Disease: Characteristics of Men Aged 40-59 in Seven Countries. *Acta Medica Scandinavica,* 460 (Supplement): 1-392.

5. Gonos, E. S. (2000). Genetics of Aging: Lessons from Centenarians. *Experimental Gerontology,* 35 (February): 15-21.

6. Pew Internet & American Life Project. Half of American Adults Have Searched Online for Health Information. Available online at <http://www.pewinternet.org/pdfs/PIP_Health_Report_July_2003.pdf>.

7. Pew Internet & American Life Project. The State of Blogging. Available online at <http://www.pewinternet.org/pdfs/PIP_blogging_data.pdf>.

Chapter 2

General Health Sites

Ask NOAH
<http://www.noah-health.org/>

New York Online Access to Health (NOAH) features content in English and Spanish languages; health topics arranged alphabetically; and health topics organized according to conditions or body systems (infections, dental care, stomach and intestines, etc.). NOAH features "full-text consumer health information that is current, relevant, accurate and unbiased."

☑ Centers for Disease Control and Prevention (CDC)
<http://www.cdc.gov/>

The CDC is a United States government agency that is devoted to health promotion and education. The site includes health and safety topics, publications and products, data and statistics, links to conferences and events, and helpful tips for staying well.

Combined Health Information Database (CHID)
<http://chid.nih.gov/>

CHID is a database of bibliographic citations related to consumer health information and education that can be searched by key words, or browsed by topics ranging from AIDS to weight control. The database is maintained by the U.S. National Institutes of Health (NIH) and is updated in January, April, July, and October.

☑ eMedicine
<http://www.emedicine.com/>
<http://www.emedicinehealth.com/>

Although this site is intended for practicing health professionals, content can be sorted according to audience (articles and continuing medical education for health professionals, and patient information for consumers), or consumers can access eMedicine Health by completing a free registration process. Site features include health resource centers ranging from asthma to mental health; lifestyle and wellness centers (emotional wellness, exercise, nutrition, weight management, men's health, outdoor living, senior health, social and family health, substance abuse, teen health, and women's health); first aid and emergencies (allergic reaction and anaphylactic shock; back, neck, and head injury; breathing difficulties; burns; cardiopulmonary resuscitation [CPR] and choking; cuts, scrapes, bruises, and blisters; diabetic coma and insulin shock; dislocations; drowning; drug overdose; fainting; fever; first aid kits; food poisoning; foreign bodies; fractures and broken bones; and more); topics arranged alphabetically from abdominal pain in adults to yoga; medical dictionary; calculators (e.g., body mass index, converting temperatures from Centigrade to Fahrenheit and Fahrenheit to Centigrade, etc.); drug recalls and alerts, and more.

Federal Citizen Information Center—Health
<http://www.pueblo.gsa.gov/health/>

The Federal Citizen Information Center in Pueblo, Colorado, is known for its distribution of pamphlets of interest and use to American consumers. The site's health section links to HTML versions of pamphlets or comsumers can request them to be mailed to a specific address. Booklet examples cover topics such as finding medical information, the use of laser surgery to erase facial wrinkles, cataracts in adults, managing chronic pain, and more.

☑ FirstGov for Consumers: Health
<http://www.consumer.gov/health.htm>

FirstGov is the U.S. government's Web portal, an aggregated interface that can be used to search for content available on federal and state government sites (see Figure 2.1). FirstGov is further subdivided into areas of in-

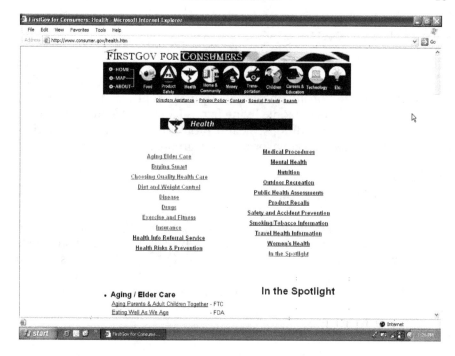

FIGURE 2.1. FirstGov for Consumers: Health
<http://www.consumer.gov/health.htm>

terest including a channel that focuses on consumer information from various government agencies. Site content on health ranges from aging/elder care to exercise and fitness to women's health.

☑ HealthAtoZ
<http://www.healthatoz.com/healthatoz/Atoz/default.jsp>

HealthAtoZ was developed by a team of health professionals including physicians, nurses, and pharmacists. Site features include channels devoted to men, women, children, and seniors; health calculators and quizzes; online personal health records; message boards; encyclopedia of health conditions; and a life clock based on lifestyle. Access requires free registration but allows for personalization based on this process.

Health Canada/Santé Canada
<http://www.hc-sc.gc.ca/>

Health Canada is Canada's federal health agency. Site content is available in English and French languages. Site features include health information for specific constituencies (aboriginal people, educators, people with disabilities, seniors, people living in rural areas, etc.); tips for healthy living; diseases and conditions; health protection; and media materials (speeches, news releases, advisories, and warnings).

☑ HealthDay
<http://www.healthday.com/>

HealthDay is a division of ScoutNews, and its main product "is a daily news feed of consumer health news stories available to media companies and a number of health-related firms, including hospitals, HMOs, health insurers, and e-health content marketers." Site features include daily news, archived news, book reviews, and content in English and Spanish languages.

Healthfinder
<http://www.healthfinder.gov/>

The National Health Information Center of the U.S. Department of Health and Human Services maintains Healthfinder as a source of authoritative health news; selected health topics; online checkups (e.g., osteoporosis risk test, recognizing hearing loss, and more); health observances (Heart Health Month, Better Sleep Month, and so forth); health news; and links to external sources of health information.

☑ HealthScout
<http://www.healthscout.com/>

HealthScout is a health portal that syndicates the use of health news, services, and tools to other sites. Portal features include channels devoted to women, men, children, seniors, diseases, addictions, sex and relationships, diet and fitness, alternative medicine, and a drug checker. The portal also includes quizzes and calculators (cholesterol, sleep, allergies, etc.), three-dimensional health animations, encyclopedia, news, more than ten special interest newsletters, and more.

InteliHealth
<http://www.intelihealth.com/>

In this site, Aetna, Inc., works with various partners (Harvard Medical School, University of Pennsylvania School of Dental Medicine) to provide access to consumer health content about diseases and conditions, healthy lifestyle, children's health, men's health, women's health, seniors' health, genetic testing, dental health, health commentaries, and more. Site features include a drug resource center; ask the expert; daily news; discussion boards; health e-mail messages; and interactive tools related to serving sizes, body mass index, and more.

MayoClinic.com
<http://www.mayoclinic.com/>

The renowned Mayo Clinic has locations in Rochester, Minnesota; Jacksonville, Florida; and Scottsdale, Arizona. The Mayo Clinic site offers authoritative consumer health information including diseases and conditions, healthy living, drug search, health tools such as calculators and quizzes, books and newsletters, and more.

Medical College of Wisconsin HealthLink
<http://healthlink.mcw.edu/>

The Medical College of Wisconsin developed HealthLink as a means to disseminate authoritative health information for consumers. Features include health news, articles browsable by topic, columns written by physicians, and ways to locate physicians and clinics and to make medical appointments.

☑ MedicineNet.com
<http://www.medicinenet.com/>

Launched in 1996, MedicineNet.com features health content developed by "over 70 U. S. board certified physicians." Site features include focused topics from allergies to women's health; diseases and conditions; symptoms and signs; procedures and tests; medications; MedTerms dictionary, e-publications, and more.

☑ MedlinePlus
<http://medlineplus.gov/>

MedlinePlus, produced by the National Library of Medicine (NLM), provides access to authoritative, full-text information on more than 650 diseases and conditions of interest to consumers and health professionals alike. Resources include a medical encyclopedia and dictionaries; downloadable health pamphlets; health information from the media; information on prescription and nonprescription drugs; directories of physicians, dentists, hospitals, and health care services; and links to external sites with reliable health content. The content is presented in the English and Spanish languages.

MedWeb
<http://www.medweb.emory.edu/MedWeb/>

The Health Sciences Center Library at Emory University in Atlanta, Georgia, developed this megasite as a means to organize Internet content about the biological and physical sciences, clinical practice, consumer health, diseases and conditions, drugs, health care, institutions, mental health, publications, and specialties.

☑ NetWellness
<http://www.netwellness.org/>

This consumer health information site represents the combined efforts of faculty affiliated with University of Cincinnati, Ohio State University, and Case Western Reserve University. Site features include ask an expert, health topics, current health news, health encyclopedia, information about clinical trials, sources of medical referrals and health providers, and more.

☑ WebMD Health
<http://my.webmd.com/>

WebMD Health includes useful content including diseases and conditions, symptoms, drugs and herbs, health tools (quizzes, calculators, self-assessments, etc.), clinical trials, health and wellness, diet and nutrition, and more. Much of the information is written by physicians and medical editors. Most of the content is free, but subscribers are entitled to individualized information and premium content such as interactive tools, newsletters, message boards, and live Web-based events with leading experts.

☑ World Health Organization (WHO)
<http://www.who.int/>

WHO is an international agency based in Geneva, Switzerland, that functions as the health agency of the United Nations (UN). Site features include health topics, publications, research tools, health statistics and health care information for UN countries, information about disease outbreaks, health information for travelers, and more.

Chapter 3

Aging and Seniors Sites

AARP Health Guide
<http://www.aarp.org/healthguide>

The American Association of Retired Persons (AARP) is a nonprofit organization that focuses on issues and concerns of Americans who are fifty years of age and older. This guide focuses on health conditions, treatments, and wellness topics; medications; medical tests; support groups; and information about Medicare coverage, low-income programs, and prescription drugs.

Ageing and Life Course
<http://www.who.int/hpr/ageing/>

The World Health Organization (WHO) in Geneva, Switzerland, developed this "course" that focuses on providing guidelines to prepare primary health centers to handle the health needs of the world's aging population. Projects of this new initiative include preventing elder abuse, teaching geriatrics to medical students, developing age-friendly standards, understanding the impact of HIV/AIDS on older persons, and more. This initiative has also established events such as the International Day of Older Persons held in October and conferences that focus on aging. The content is available in English, French, and Spanish languages.

Division of Aging and Seniors
<http://www.phac-aspc.gc.ca/seniors-aines>

Canada's Division of Aging and Seniors "provides federal leadership in areas pertaining to aging and seniors," including information and expertise. Site features include a calendar of events, press releases, publications, and links to external sites. Content is featured in English and French languages.

ElderWeb
<http://www.elderweb.com/>

ElderWeb was developed in 1994 by Karen Stevenson, a certified public accountant and "consultant with over 19 years of experience in long term care, finance, and technology." Site features focus on long-term care and include news, book reviews, events, glossary, search of U.S. government documents, links to statistics, finance and law, housing and care, and more. Text font size can be made larger or smaller, and colors can be changed for better contrast and readability.

GrowYouthful.com
<http://www.growyouthful.com/>

The companion Web site to David Niven Miller's *Grow Youthful* book includes a biological age test, body mass index calculator, excerpts from the book, recipes, top anti-aging tips, and more (see Figure 3.1).

Health—Senior Health
<http://www.emedicinehealth.com/collections/SU313.asp>

eMedicine is a site intended for health professionals that also includes useful consumer health information which requires free registration. The section about senior health includes subsections devoted to cholesterol, circulation problems, dementia, glaucoma, heart, and stroke; articles about advance directives, end-of-life decisions, hearing loss, joint replacement, macular degeneration, menopause, and other topics; and common health tests (see Figure 3.2). Additional site information includes a medical dictionary, drug recalls and alerts, and useful tools for calculating ideal weight, body mass index, and more.

☑ HealthScout: Seniors
<http://www.healthscout.com/channel/1/1001/main.html>

HealthScout is a health portal that syndicates the use of health news, services, and tools to other sites. The channel devoted to seniors includes

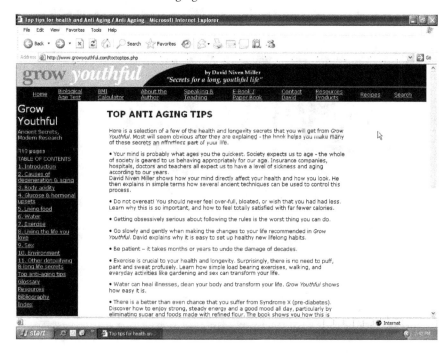

FIGURE 3.1. GrowYouthful.com—Top Anti-Aging Tips
<http://www.growyouthful.com/toctoptips.php>
Used with permission by GrowYouthful.com.

health-related video clips (treatments for back pain, medical conditions related to aging for persons fifty years of age and older, laser therapy for macular degeneration, and more), news articles, drug information, and more.

☑ Healthy Aging for Older Adults
<http://www.cdc.gov/aging/>

The U.S. Centers for Disease Control and Prevention (CDC) site includes information about "promoting health, preventing disease, and enhancing quality of life among older Americans." Features include information about health-related behaviors, chronic diseases, infectious diseases, adult immunizations, injuries in adults, Medicare, and more.

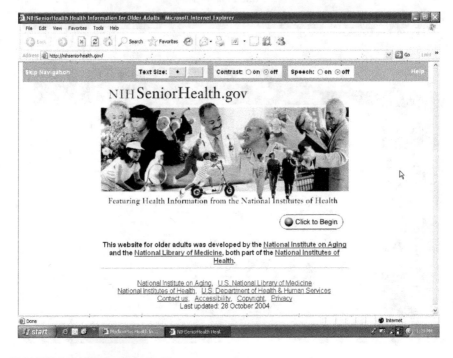

FIGURE 3.2. NIH Senior Health.gov
<http://nihseniorhealth.gov/>

☑ Infoaging.org
<http://www.infoaging.org/>

The American Federation for Aging Research (AFAR) developed this
site with funding from Pfizer Inc., the pharmaceutical company (see Figure 3.3). The site focuses on three major areas: biology of aging, disease
center, and healthy aging. The biology of aging section includes information about antioxidants, biomarkers, theories of aging, caloric restriction,
stem cells, animal models of aging, and more. The disease center covers
basic information about Alzheimer's disease, breast cancer, depression,
diabetes, heart diseases, macular degeneration, osteoarthritis, osteoporosis, prostate cancer, and stroke, and how each relates to aging. The healthy
aging section focuses on lifestyle including nutrition, exercise, sleep,
stress, alcohol, smoking cessation, vision, hearing, oral health, and immunization. Other special features include news, research, ask the expert, and
Lifelong, a series of publications available free in print or by e-mail.

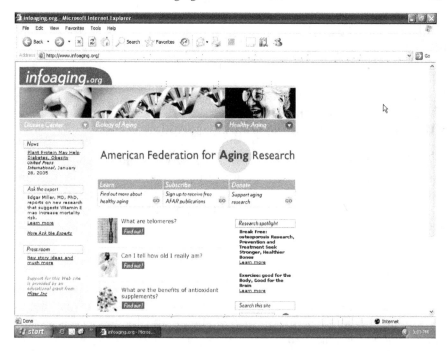

FIGURE 3.3. Infoaging.org
<http://www.infoaging.org/>
Used with permission by the American Federation for Aging Research.

Institute of Gerontology
<http://www.iog.wayne.edu/>

Wayne State University's Institute of Gerontology (IOG) site features text and a Web broadcast of the "Tips on Aging Well" radio segment hosted by Bob Allison on WNZK 690 AM, events calendar, and e-mail versions of the IOG Transitions Online publication.

MayoClinic.com—Senior Health Center
<http://www.mayoclinic.com/>

The renowned Mayo Clinic has locations in Rochester, Minnesota; Jacksonville, Florida; and Scottsdale, Arizona. Senior Health is one of more than twenty-five health centers developed by the Mayo Clinic on its consumer health site. Features include an aging quiz, information about screening tests, health issues of interest to aging adults, and tips for staying sharp mentally, living a long and healthy life, and maintaining independence.

Medical College of Wisconsin HealthLink
<http://aging.healthlink.mcw.edu/>
<http://healthlink.mcw.edu/aging/index.html>

The Medical College of Wisconsin organizes this information into two parts on HealthLink. Features include articles about memory loss, living with chronic diseases, advance directives, nutrition after menopause, loss of taste and smell due to specific medications, advice for aging athletes, and more.

NIHSeniorHealth
<http://nihseniorhealth.gov/>

This U.S. government site was developed by the National Institute on Aging and the National Library of Medicine and focuses on aspects of senior health including Alzheimer's disease, arthritis, balance problems, breast cancer, colorectal cancer, diabetes, exercise for older adults, hearing loss, lung cancer, prostate cancer, and taking medications (see Figure 3.2). Special site features include increasing/decreasing text size, increasing/decreasing site contrast, and activating/deactivating speech. Users have the option of reading or hearing text contained on this site.

Online Mendelian Inheritance in Man (OMIM)
<http://www.ncbi.nlm.nih.gov/entrez/query.fcgi?=OMIM>

This site is a database that includes descriptions, citations, and genetic information about a wide array of diseases, medical conditions, and physiological processes. The information refers to research studies about genetic mutations that can contribute to physical signs of aging.

SeniorHealthCare.org
<http://www.seniorhealthcare.org/>

SeniorHealthCare is a site with content developed by nurses and physicians, some of whom are affiliated with Union Memorial Hospital in Baltimore. Site features include calendar of events; "Senior Expressions," which is a site section that encourages seniors to write and share their thoughts; Ask the Experts; hot health topics which includes alcoholism, dementia, hospice care, sleep disorders, incontinence, and more; electronic newsletter issues; Webcasts; news about geriatrics research; legislation and health care policies that affect seniors; and more.

SeniorNavigator.com
<http://www.seniornavigator.com/>

SeniorNavigator.com is a not-for-profit organization that refers to itself as "Virginia's Resource for Health and Aging." Site features include a community calendar, Ask an Expert, a free online class that trains SeniorNavigator volunteers, a neighborhood discussion forum, finding health services by zip code, and more. Free registration allows for customization of content including saving articles or links in "My Library" and interacting with the site's volunteer experts.

☑ **Seniors' Health Issues**
<http://www.nlm.nih.gov/medlineplus/seniorshealthissues.html>

MedlinePlus is a consumer health resource developed by the U.S. National Library of Medicine that provides extensive information about more than 650 diseases and conditions. The information about seniors' health includes an alphabetical list of health topics ranging from age-related macular degeneration to wrinkles. Other issues of concern to seniors include latest news, overviews, anatomy/physiology, clinical trials, research, prevention/screening, directories, organizations, statistics, and more (see Figure 3.4).

ThirdAge Health
<http://www.thirdage.com/health/>

This site is intended for persons in their thirties, forties, and fifties who are interested in personal growth and development. Site sections include health, relationship, money, work, beauty, fun, and food. Site features include newsletters, chat room, and discussion boards on a variety of related topics, free online classes, health quizzes, and more.

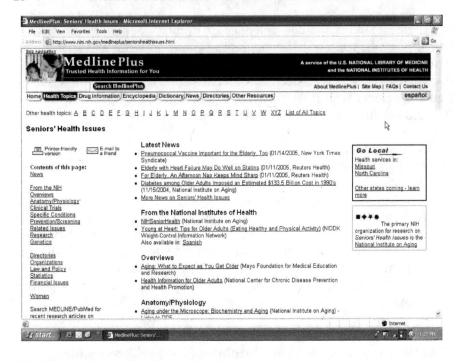

FIGURE 3.4. MedlinePlus Seniors' Health Issues
<http://www.nlm.nih.gov/medlineplus/seniorshealthissues.html>

Chapter 4

Anti-Aging and Longevity Sites

Ageless Forever
<http://www.agelessforever.net/qanda.asp>

Ageless Forever is an anti-aging and longevity center based in Las Vegas, Nevada. The center's site features information about theories, supplements, nutrition, hormones, exercise, products, asking the doctor questions, glossary, and articles.

☑ Aging 101
<http://www.hcoa.org/aging/intro.htm>

The Huffington Center on Aging (HCOA) at Baylor College of Medicine in Houston, Texas, focuses on many aspects of aging research including centenarians, secretagogues, cognitive function, neurodegenerative diseases, tumor suppressor genes, and more. Site content includes chapters about the mysteries, processes, psychology, demographics, and genetics of aging.

☑ Anti-Aging Guide
<http://www.anti-aging-guide.com/>

This cluttered, colorful, and busy site was developed by Arcady L. Economo who holds doctoral degrees (including one in pharmacy), and is associated with Anti-Aging Europe Fasting and Cleansing Program <http://www.antiaging-europe.com>. Site sections include fasting and calorie restriction, anti-aging nutrition, anti-aging drugs and supplements, quality of life, and exercise and physical activity. The outlined content is thorough and supplemented with news articles, research article abstracts, products, information about conferences, database of nutrients, discussion forum, and more (see Figure 4.1).

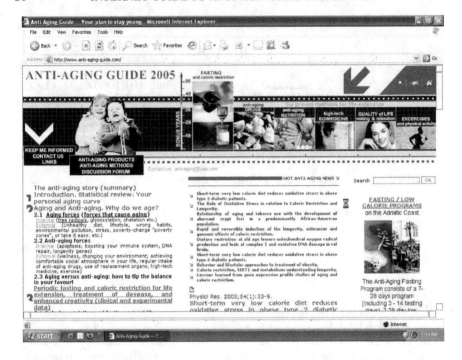

FIGURE 4.1. Anti-Aging Guide
<http://www.anti-aging-guide.com/>
Used with permission.

Anti-Aging Medicine
<http://www.anti-agingmd.com/antiaging.html>

Clif Arrington is a Hawaii-based physician who is interested in anti-aging medicine. His site includes information about dehydroepiandrosterone (DHEA), human growth hormone, male menopause, testosterone treatment, chelation therapy, hormone testing, immune support, oxidative therapy, and other treatments.

Anti-Aging Strategies
<http://www.drlam.com/anti-agingstratagiesbrief.cfm>

Dr. Michael Lam is a physician who specializes in nutrition and anti-aging. His site groups anti-aging strategies into five categories: diet, exercise, hormonal enhancement, nutritional supplements, and stress reduction. Site information includes protocols, his opinions, news, archived news, and more.

☑ Anti-Aging-Research.US
<http://www.anti-aging-research.us/>

Anti-Aging-Research.US is a public information project sponsored by Medaus, a manufacturer of pharmacy solutions. Site content includes theories on aging, declining biological processes, hormone therapy, optimal nutrition, and more. The site's Anti-Aging Resource Center features articles, news headlines, and streaming video clips about the effects of aging, gene therapy, hormone replacement therapy, and related topics.

Center for Healthy Aging
<http://www.centerforhealthyaging.org/>

Located in Los Angeles, the Center for Healthy Aging is a nonprofit organization that was founded in 1976 "to meet the needs of aging adults and their families." Site features include calendar of events, training, programs and services, resources, and news.

Health and Age
<http://www.healthandage.com>

Health and Age's motto is "live well, live longer" and "is sponsored by the Web-based Health Education Foundation (WHEF), an independent non-profit organization," although the site was created originally "by the Novartis Foundation for Gerontology in 1998." Site features include news, articles, disease digests, tools, newsletter, publications including *Primer on Geriatrics,* and links to government information about aging. The site is also organized into information for caregivers, men's health, and women's health. Users can adjust content font size from normal-point type to large or extra large.

Healthful Life Project
<http://healthfullife.umdnj.edu/index.htm>

The Healthful Life Project publishes a newsletter about living a healthier life and promotes a Health-Full-Life Program that recommends specific tests, comprehensive prevention physical examination, and a series of lifestyle changes that focus on good nutrition, weight control, regular exercise, and nonsmoking.

HealthWorld Online – Healthy Aging Center
<http://www.healthy.net/scr/center.asp?centerid=3>

HealthWorld Online is managed by a physician director and an advisory board of physicians, nurses, scientists, and other health professionals. Site features of the Healthy Aging Center include news, updates, information about alternative therapies (herbs, qigong, nutrition), related conditions (Alzheimer's disease, senile dementia, baldness, macular degeneration, etc.), and more.

Healthy Aging Center
<http://www.healthyaging.net/>

Healthy Aging Center is "the official site of the Healthy Aging Campaign—a national ongoing health promotion designed to broaden awareness of the positive aspects of aging and to provide information and inspiration for adults, age 50+, to improve their physical, mental, social, and financial fitness," as developed by Educational Television Network, Inc., of Unionville, Pennsylvania. Site features include a calendar of events related to aging; ordering information for books, videos, and educational materials related to the subject; free tips and techniques about physical, mental, social, and financial aspects of aging that can be used in educational handouts developed by others; and links to external aging sites.

☑ Healthy Aging for Older Adults
<http://www.cdc.gov/aging/>

The U.S. Centers for Disease Control and Prevention (CDC) site includes health information for older adults that covers health-related behaviors, chronic diseases, infectious diseases, immunizations for adults, injuries among older adults, Medicare, and more; health statistics and research related to aging; links to federal government organizations related to the subject as well as other organizations; publications; and an electronic forum for discussing these issues (see Figure 4.2).

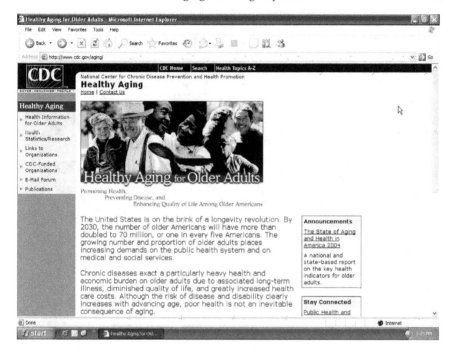

FIGURE 4.2. Healthy Aging for Older Adults
<http://www.cdc.gov/aging/>

Healthy Aging Partnership
<http://www.4elders.org/>

Although Healthy Aging Partnership is intended for older citizens living in King, Kitsap, Pierce, and Snohomish counties in the Puget Sound region of Washington State, the partnership's site includes useful information about healthy living (detecting and preventing elder abuse, the importance of a varied diet, preventing heart attacks, understanding food labels, and more); and links about aging for seniors and caregivers of seniors.

☑ Longevity Meme
<http://www.longevitymeme.org>

This site focuses on three main messages: live healthily, fight aging, and extend your life (see Figure 4.3). The term "meme" means a behavioral

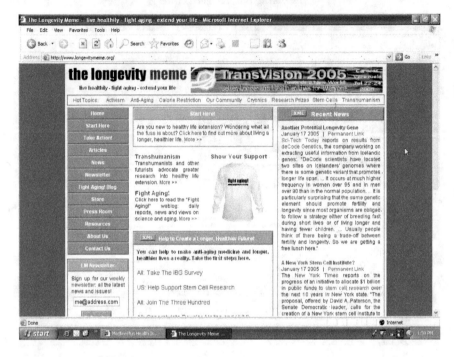

FIGURE 4.3. Longevity Meme
<http://www.longevitymeme.org/>
Used with permission by Longevity Meme.

value that is passed from one generation to another by means of imitation. The site defines itself as "the collection of ideas, viewpoints and behaviors that will enable people to lead long, healthy and extended lives." Site features include hot topics (activism, anti-aging, calorie restriction, cryonics, stem cells, transhumanism); informative articles; news; newsletter; blog; calendar of events; online store of longevity merchandise; funding sources; and more.

Longevity Science
<http://longevity-science.org/>

Calling itself a scientific and educational Web site on human longevity, this site's stated purpose is "to understand the mechanisms of aging and longevity to extend healthy and productive human lifespan." The site developers are Leonid A. Gavrilov and Natalia S. Gavrilova, researchers at the Center on Aging at the University of Chicago. Site features include news, articles (some written by Gavrilov and Gavrilova), links to external sites, and more.

Methuselah Mouse Prize
<http://www.methuselahmouse.org/>

The Methuselah Foundation will award money "to the scientific research team who develops the longest living *Mus musculus,* the breed of mouse most commonly used in scientific research." The thinking is that the same techniques that are used to breed this mouse can be used to extend life spans in humans. Site features include news information about rejuvenation, documents to help raise funds for this cause, details for researchers interested in competing, links to other sites, and more.

☑ RealAge
<http://www.realage.com/>

RealAge's premise is that is it possible to look younger and live longer by paying attention to family history, diet, exercise, existing health conditions, personal habits, and other factors (see Figure 4.4). Site features include a test that helps determine a person's "real age"—meaning the physiological age of the body based on various factors, diet and health tools, exercise plans, personalized health information and assessments, daily tips, and more. Free registration allows for customization of information, scoring of health quizzes, and access to most site information. Premium members pay a monthly fee to access *RealAge Report,* bonus materials about avoiding diseases, and personalized recommendations for looking and feeling younger.

☑ SAGE Crossroads
<http://www.sagecrossroads.net/public/>

This is an online forum devoted to the subject of human aging that is funded by the Ellison Medical Foundation and the American Association for the Advancement of Science (AAAS). Site features include news and opinions about "aging-related research and policy," live online debates that

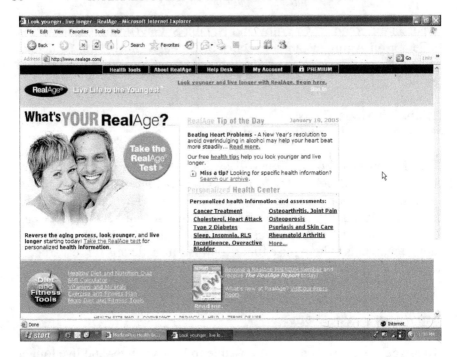

FIGURE 4.4. RealAge
<http://www.realage.com/>
Used with permission.

feature experts discussing topics that range from longevity to bioethics, and a video archive of past Webcasts (see Figure 4.5).

☑ World Health Network
<http://www.worldhealth.net/>

The American Academy of Anti-Aging Medicine (A4M), with more than 12,500 physicians and scientists as members, is a nonprofit, professional organization that "is dedicated to the advancement of technology to detect, prevent, and treat aging related disease and to promote research into methods to retard and optimize the human aging process." A4M's WorldHealth.net site includes news; newsletter; directory of physicians, clinics, products, and spas; information about conferences; top twenty articles about anti-aging; information about theories on aging; and more.

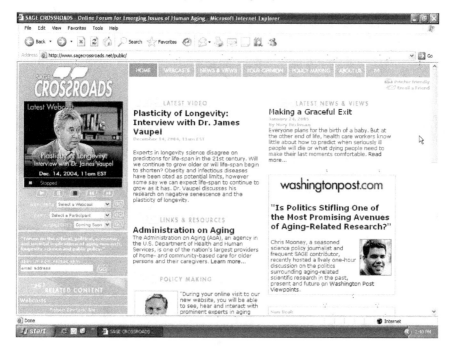

FIGURE 4.5. SAGE Crossroads
<http://www.sagecrossroads.net/public/>
Used with permission by Alliance for Aging Research.

Chapter 5

Diseases and Conditions of Aging

The essence of life is statistical improbability on a colossal scale.

Richard Dawkins

BONE AND JOINT CONDITIONS

Aging Changes in the Bones—Muscles—Joints
<http://health.allrefer.com/health/aging-changes-in-the-bones-muscles-joints-info.html>

AllRefer.com is a megasite that is organized into an encyclopedia, gazetteer, and four main channels: health, yellow pages, reference, and weather. Within the health channel, the information about aging changes in the bones, muscles, and joints includes pictures and images, explanation of common problems (osteoporosis, muscle weakness, gait changes, tremors, etc.), prevention, and related topics.

Arthritis (MedlinePlus)
<http://www.nlm.nih.gov/medlineplus/arthritis.html>

MedlinePlus is a consumer health resource developed by the U.S. National Library of Medicine that provides extensive information about more than 650 diseases and conditions. The information about arthritis includes latest news, overviews, anatomy/physiology, diagnosis/symptoms, treatment, health check tools, clinical trials, alternative therapy, nutrition, disease management, coping, rehabilitation, research, directories, organizations, statistics, financial issues, and arthritis in women or children.

Bone Diseases (MedlinePlus)
<http://www.nlm.nih.gov/medlineplus/bonediseases.html>

MedlinePlus is a consumer health resource developed by the U.S. National Library of Medicine that provides extensive information about more than 650 diseases and conditions. The information about bone diseases includes anatomy/physiology, diagnosis/symptoms, treatment, clinical trials, prevention/screening, genetics, directories, organizations, statistics, and bone diseases in children.

Hip Replacement (MedlinePlus)
<http://www.nlm.nih.gov/medlineplus/hipreplacement.html>

MedlinePlus is a consumer health resource developed by the U.S. National Library of Medicine that provides extensive information about more than 650 diseases and conditions. The information about hip replacement includes overviews, pictures/diagrams, rehabilitation, research, directories, and organizations.

Knee Replacement (MedlinePlus)
<http://www.nlm.nih.gov/medlineplus/kneereplacement.html>

MedlinePlus is a consumer health resource developed by the U.S. National Library of Medicine that provides extensive information about more than 650 diseases and conditions. The information about knee replacement includes overviews, clinical trials, rehabilitation, research, directories, organizations, and newsletters/print publications.

Osteoarthritis Center (RealAge Arthritis Center)
<http://www.realage.com/health_guides/osteoarthritis/introduction. asp>

RealAge's premise is that is it possible to look younger and live longer by paying attention to family history, diet, exercise, existing health conditions, personal habits, and other factors. The center devoted to arthritis and joint pain relief includes information about symptoms, diet and nutrition, exercise, medication, treatment, natural remedies, and more.

Osteoporosis (MedicineNet)
<http://www.medicinenet.com/osteoporosis/article.htm>

Launched in 1996, MedicineNet.com features health content developed by "over 70 U.S. board certified physicians." The information on osteoporosis includes definition, symptoms, risk factors, diagnostic tests, treatment, prevention, future research, and more.

Osteoporosis (MedlinePlus)
<http://www.nlm.nih.gov/medlineplus/osteoporosis.html>

MedlinePlus is a consumer health resource developed by the U.S. National Library of Medicine that provides extensive information about more than 650 diseases and conditions. The information about osteoporosis includes latest news, overviews, anatomy/physiology, diagnosis/symptoms, health check tools, clinical trials, prevention/screening, nutrition, disease management, coping, research, organizations, statistics, and osteoporosis in women, men, children, or teenagers.

GENERAL CONDITIONS

Aging Gracefully
<http://www.pioneerthinking.com/lmc-aging.html>

Pioneer Thinking focuses on mind and body, home and family, and lifestyle. The information about aging gracefully was written by a "licensed aesthetician and registered dietetic technician." Recommendations include healthy eating, especially foods that include specific vitamins and minerals that help keep the skin youthful and fresh, avoiding or reducing sun exposure, using skin cleansers and moisturizers, and other healthy habits. Site content can be translated from English to French, German, Italian, Japanese, Chinese, Russian, Spanish, or Swedish.

Aging Successfully
<http://centeronaging.uams.edu/doctor_david/aging_successfully.
  asp>

The Donald W. Reynolds Center on Aging at the University of Arkansas for Medical Sciences funded a twenty-six-part television series about aging titled *Aging Successfully with Doctor David,* hosted by Dr. David Lipschitz. This series was shown on Arkansas Educational Television Network (AETN) and has been licensed to run on PBS. This site features an episode guide with video clips. Topics include positive effects of good lifestyle choices, nutrition, exercise, health screenings, memory loss, death and dying, frailty, vitamins and minerals, creativity and aging, sexuality and aging, and more.

☑ Aging: What to Expect As You Get Older (Mayo Clinic)
<http://www.mayoclinic.com/invoke.cfm?id=HA00040>

The renowned Mayo Clinic has locations in Rochester, Minnesota; Jacksonville, Florida; and Scottsdale, Arizona. Its consumer health site information about aging explains natural changes in the cardiovascular system; bones and joints; digestive system; kidneys and urinary tract; brain and nervous system; eyes, ears, teeth, and skin; nails and hair; sleep; weight; sexuality; and ways to live a healthier lifestyle.

Biomarkers of Aging Information Center (AFAR)
<http://www.infoaging.org/b-biomark-2-what.html>

The American Federation for Aging Research (AFAR) developed this site with funding from Pfizer Inc., the pharmaceutical company. The site focuses on three major areas: biology of aging, disease center, and healthy aging. The information about biomarkers of aging describes research into aging and interventions that may slow the process, and links to current research about cell replication rate, hormonal changes, and immunological measurements that may serve as possible biomarkers of aging.

The Facets of Aging
<http://www.sos.mo.gov/library/development/services/seniors/manual/ch1.pdf>

The Missouri State Library developed this fifteen-page document which outlines age-related changes affecting vision, hearing, taste, smell, and dexterity which need to be taken into consideration when planning library services for older adults. The document also discusses myths and stereotypes about aging; eighteen principles related to independence, participation, care, self-fulfillment, and dignity adopted by the General Assembly of the United Nations to guide interactions with older persons; and the importance of lifelong learning.

Keeping That Get Up and Go
<http://www.rehabpub.com/features/32001/2.asp>

Rehab Management is a publication that focuses on "recent advances in the rehabilitation marketplace along with news and current issues in the rehab industry." The journal's site includes free information about the benefits of exercising to reduce mobility disorders, especially among seniors.

HAIR LOSS

Causes of Hair Loss
<http://www.afraidtoask.com/hair/causesofhairloss.html>

Afraidtoask.com was developed by a Rhode Island physician to address health issues that people may be timid to talk or ask about such as sexually transmitted diseases, pubic hair, genitalia, and other subjects. This illustrated and animated information covers patterns of male and female baldness, sudden hair loss, and other forms of partial or complete baldness.

Hair Diseases and Hair Loss
<http://www.nlm.nih.gov/medlineplus/hairdiseasesandhairloss.html>

MedlinePlus is a consumer health resource developed by the U.S. National Library of Medicine that provides extensive information about more than 650 diseases and conditions. The information about hair loss includes overviews; diagnosis/symptoms; treatment; clinical trials; specific hair conditions; organizations; statistics; hair loss in women, men, children, or teenagers; and more. The content is available in English and Spanish languages.

Hair Loss in Men and Women
<http://www.medicinenet.com/hair_loss/article.htm>

Launched in 1996, MedicineNet.com features health content developed by "over 70 U.S. board certified physicians." The information about hair loss includes causes and treatments, and how hair loss differs in men and women.

Symptom: Hair Symptoms (Wrong Diagnosis)
<http://www.wrongdiagnosis.com/sym/hair_symptoms.htm>

This site was developed by patients who sought useful, factual information about various diseases and health conditions. The section on hair symptoms includes information about diseases, conditions, and deficiencies that can affect the hair.

HEARING LOSS

Age-Related Hearing Loss
<http://www.nlm.nih.gov/medlineplus/ency/article/001045.htm>

This brief encyclopedic entry for age-related hearing loss includes alternative names (presbycusis), definition, causes, symptoms, tests, treatment, prognosis, complications, and more.

Defeating Deafness
<http://www.defeatingdeafness.org/?lid=1619>

Defeating Deafness (The Hearing Research Trust) is a United Kingdom-based charity that seeks to cure and/or prevent deafness. The information about age-related hearing loss includes an explanation of the degenerative processes that can lead to partial or total deafness, research developments, and news and media reports.

Difference Between Deaf and Hard of Hearing (NAD)
<http://www.nad.org/site/pp.asp?c=foINKQMBF&b=180410>

The National Association of the Deaf (NAD) site explains the terms deaf, Deaf, and hard of hearing (mild to moderate loss of hearing); includes information about American Sign Language, captioning of media programming, advocacy issues, education, and more.

Hearing Loss in Adults
<http://www.intelihealth.com/IH/ihtIH/WSIHW000/9339/9418. html>

Aetna, Inc., works with Harvard Medical School to provide access to consumer health content about diseases and conditions including this information about age-related hearing loss (definition, symptoms, diagnosis, expected duration, prevention, treatment, when to call a professional, prognosis, and additional information).

INCONTINENCE

Fecal Incontinence
<http://familydoctor.org/067.xml>

The American Academy of Family Physicians provides this information about "the loss of normal control of the bowels," which can occur at any age. Details include a definition, an explanation of the causes, testing, and treatments. The information is available in English and Spanish languages.

Incontinence: An Overview
<http://www.seekwellness.com/incontinence/index.htm>

This overview of urinary incontinence on the SeekWellness site was written by a nurse. Information includes questions to determine whether someone has a bladder control problem, a publication titled *Report of a Survey of Women with Bladder Control Problems,* a downloadable poster, and a color brochure on the same subject.

Urinary Incontinence (MedicineNet)
<http://www.medicinenet.com/urinary_incontinence/article.htm>

Launched in 1996, MedicineNet.com features health content developed by "over 70 U.S. board certified physicians." The information about loss of urinary control includes causes, types, treatments, and more.

Urinary Incontinence (MedlinePlus)
<http://www.nlm.nih.gov/medlineplus/urinaryincontinence.html>

MedlinePlus is a consumer health resource developed by the U.S. National Library of Medicine that provides extensive information about more than 650 diseases and conditions. The information about loss of urinary control includes overviews, anatomy/physiology, diagnosis/symptoms, treatment, clinical trials, coping, directories, organizations, and more.

MEMORY

Memory and Aging: Improving Your Memory (Helpguide)
<http://www.helpguide.org/life/improving_memory.htm>

Helpguide is "Expert, non-commercial information on mental health and lifelong wellness: A project of the Rotary Club of Santa Monica and Center for Healthy Aging." The information about memory and aging covers ways to improve memory; registration, retention, and recall as the three components of memory; tools and tactics (writing notes, designing living environments to reduce frustration, and using physical cues as reminders); importance of imagery, association, and organization to retention; and links to external sites about memory.

Memory in the Aging Brain (Virtual Hospital)
<http://www.vh.org/adult/provider/neurology/memory/>

Virtual Hospital, "a digital library of health information," provides brief information about age-related mental decline including loss of acuity and memory written by Steven W. Anderson, PhD, and Dr. Thomas J. Grabowski.

Memory Loss and Aging
<http://www.aarp.org/nrta/Articles/a2003-08-19-memoryloss.html>

This information is part of AARP's Staying Sharp Series which focuses on several topics related to aging including memory loss, cognitive fitness, chronic diseases, depression, and lifelong learning. The ten-page document about memory loss covers normal forgetfulness, brain research into memory, tips for staying sharp (relax, concentrate, focus, slow down, organize, write it down, repeat it, and visualize it), symptoms of Alzheimer's disease, and more.

Secrets of Aging
<http://www.secretsofaging.org/mind/>

The Museum of Science in Boston, Massachusetts, featured an exhibit about the secrets of aging. The exhibit site includes video clips of Art Buchwald, Betty Friedan, and Maya Angelou who talk about Social Security, growing older, and friendship, respectively; the site also includes interactive tools that test intelligence, contextual memory, memory grouping, misconceptions about aging; and more.

MENOPAUSE/ANDROPAUSE

Ageing Male Syndrome
<http://www.4woman.gov/mens/print-men.cfm?page=426&mtitle= Ageing percent20Male percent20Syndrome>

The National Women's Health Information Center maintains a Web site and toll-free call center as sources of information about women's health, and to a lesser degree, men's health.

Andropause
<http://www.andropause.com/>

Andropause or male menopause refers to an age-related drop in testosterone levels. This site is maintained by NV Organon, a Netherlands-based pharmaceutical company that sells testosterone replacement therapy and other medications. Site information includes diagnosis, treatment options, tips for talking with a physician, a ten-question andropause quiz, and other resources.

Male Menopause
<http://www.clevelandclinic.org/health/health-info/docs/3000/3001.
  asp?index=10094>

This site, sponsored by the Cleveland Clinic, includes useful information on a variety of diseases and conditions. The information about the effects of declining hormone levels in men discusses diagnosis and treatment.

Menopause (eMedicine)
<http://www.emedicinehealth.com/Articles/6759-1.asp>

eMedicine is a site intended for health professionals that also includes useful consumer health information which requires free registration. The information about menopause includes an overview, causes, symptoms, when to consult a physician, examinations and tests, treatments, and more.

Menopause (MedlinePlus)
<http://www.nlm.nih.gov/medlineplus/menopause.html>

MedlinePlus is a consumer health resource developed by the U.S. National Library of Medicine that provides extensive information about more than 650 diseases and conditions. The information about menopause includes latest news, overviews, diagnosis/symptoms, treatment, clinical trials, alternative therapies, coping, research, directories, organizations, and more.

Menopause (Third Age)
<http://www.thirdage.com/health/women/>

This site is intended for persons in their thirties, forties, and fifties who are interested in personal growth and development. The information about menopause includes a quiz that tests myths and facts about the subject, decisions to take hormone replacement therapy, common symptoms, live chat about the subject, and more.

Menopause and Bladder Control
<http://kidney.niddk.nih.gov/kudiseases/pubs/menopause_ez/>

The National Kidney and Urologic Diseases Information Clearing-house (NKUDIC) is a service of the National Institute of Diabetes and Digestive and Kidney Diseases (NIDDK), which in turn in part of the U.S. National Institutes of Health (NIH). The information explains how hormonal changes related to menopause can affect bladder control, other causes of urinary incontinence, treatments, and more.

Menopause and Menopause Treatments
<http://www.4woman.gov/faq/menopaus.htm>

The National Women's Health Information Center maintains a Web site and toll-free call center as sources of information about women's health. Part of the U.S. Department of Health and Human Services, 4woman.gov provides health news, articles, a section on menopause and hormone therapy, newsletters, tools (recommended screening tests by age group, common diagnostic tests, symptoms of serious diseases, and more), dictionaries, journal articles, and more. The information about menopause includes symptoms, risks and benefits of hormone therapy, natural treatments, related conditions, and more.

SKIN CONDITIONS

Go Ask Alice! Skin Remedies
<http://www.goaskalice.columbia.edu/1655.html>

Go Ask Alice! provides answers to health questions and is hosted on Columbia University's site, which also archives more than 3,000 answered questions for the past ten years. Alice is the health education program of the university's division of Health Services. The information about skin remedies discusses the effects of sun and smoking cigarettes, importance of using sunscreen products and moisturizers, and other advice.

☑ Health Effects of Overexposure to the Sun
<http://www.epa.gov/sunwise/uvandhealth.html>

The U.S. Environmental Protection Agency's SunWise program offers this information about ultraviolet light radiation and the health effects of sun exposure, including cancer (basal cell carcinoma, melanoma, squamous cell carcinoma), premature aging, cataracts and other eye disorders, and a suppressed immune system. The site also includes brochures, posters, fact sheets, and other publications in HTML and PDF form.

Health Watch—Younger Skin
<http://www8.utsouthwestern.edu/utsw/cda/dept16498/files/144551. html>

The University of Texas Southwestern Medical Center at Dallas provides Health Watch, a public service that provides consumer health information related to the human body, special health issues (smoking, vitamins and minerals, surgery, etc.), diseases and conditions including cancer, diabetes, infectious diseases, etc., and lifetime health care for all age groups, including seniors. The information about younger skin covers the importance of using sunscreen products to prevent skin damage that leads to wrinkles.

☑ Skin Aging
<http://www.nlm.nih.gov/medlineplus/skinaging.html>

MedlinePlus is a consumer health resource developed by the U.S. National Library of Medicine that provides extensive information about more than 650 diseases and conditions. The information about skin aging includes overviews, pictures/diagrams, treatment, specific conditions (aging eyelids, liver spots on hands, etc.), research, directories, organizations, and more.

Skin Care
<http://www.healthfinder.gov/Scripts/SearchContext.asp? topic=794>

The National Health Information Center of the U.S. Department of Health and Human Services maintains Healthfinder as a source of authoritative health information from other sources. The links related to skin care include annotated links to external sources of information, and related organizations.

Skin Wrinkles
<http://www.umm.edu/patiented/articles/what_causes_wrinkles_000021_1.htm>

The University of Maryland Medical Center (UMM) site provides patient education information including this article about who is most likely to have wrinkles, relationship of the aging process to the development of wrinkles, role of sunlight in the development of wrinkles, and treatments that can reduce wrinkles.

VISION LOSS

Age-Related Macular Degeneration (Wrong Diagnosis)
<http://www.wrongdiagnosis.com/a/age_related_macular_degeneration/intro.htm>

This site was developed by patients who sought useful, factual information about various diseases and health conditions. The information about age-related macular degeneration includes a basic summary, prevalence and incidence of the disease, prognosis, risk factors, symptoms, diagnostic tests, complications, associated conditions, treatments, research, statistics, and more.

The Aging Eye
<http://agingeye.com/>

This site has a disclaimer stating that its content is intended for Canadian residents only. The site's editor in chief is a medical doctor. Two versions of the site content are presented: one with enlarged text and simplified design for visually impaired users, and the other with "standard form" for text size and site design, but the font size can be increased at any time. Site content includes information about how the eye works; diseases such as macular degeneration, diabetic retinopathy, cataracts, glaucoma, age-related maculopathy, and eye diseases not associated with age; nutrition; eye research and clinical trials; dealing with vision loss; services that ophthalmologists, optometrists, and opticians provide; preventing eye injuries; assistive technology for persons with visual impairments; and more.

Eye Health As You Grow Older
<http://www.hmc.psu.edu/healthinfo/articles/aging/eye.pdf>

This colorfully illustrated, one-page guide briefly explains age-related eye problems including presbyopia, floaters, cataracts, glaucoma, macular degeneration, and diabetic retinopathy; it recommends visual screening and describes what happens during eye examinations. This document is a Patient Page from the February 16, 2000, issue of *The Journal of the American Medical Association,* and is intended for use as consumer health information for patients interested in eye health.

The Four Most Common Causes of Age-Related Vision Loss
<http://www.visionconnection.org/Content/YourVision/
   TheAgingEye/TheFourMostCommonCausesofAgeRelatedVision
   Loss.htm>

The VisionConnection site was established by Lighthouse International and the Royal National Institute for the Blind with funding from Pfizer Ophthalmics. The site features a large font and information about prevention of vision loss, vision rehabilitation, and technology to assist with vision loss. The information about age-related vision loss refers to four major causes: macular degeneration, glaucoma, cataracts, and diabetic retinopathy, and explains each, defines low vision, describes presbyopia (normal changes in the eye due to aging), and more.

Research Focuses on Age-Related Macular Degeneration
<http://healthlink.mcw.edu/article/1031002225.html>

The Medical College of Wisconsin's HealthLink's information about macular degeneration related to age covers the difference between "wet" and "dry" forms of the condition, research into the role that melanin, antioxidants, and growth factors play in the course of the disease, and nutrients that may reduce risk of vision loss.

Chapter 6

Effects on Length of Life

ALCOHOLISM AND ALCOHOL CONSUMPTION

Aging and Alcohol Abuse
<http://www.ext.colostate.edu/pubs/consumer/10250.pdf>

This six-page document, developed by the Colorado State University Cooperative Extension and written by a gerontologist, describes the risk of alcohol abuse in aging populations. The document describes factors that contribute to alcoholism, includes a brief quiz for determining whether an older person has a problem with alcohol, and offers tips for seeking help.

Alcohol and Health
<http://www2.potsdam.edu/alcohol-info/AlcoholAndHealth.html>

This alcohol information site is hosted by the Sociology department at the State University of New York at Potsdam. The site includes information about the link between moderate drinking and longer life spans, other health benefits of moderate drinking, history of medicinal properties of alcohol, and more.

Alcohol and Health: Current Evidence
<http://www.bu.edu/act/alcoholandhealth/index.html>

Boston University publishes *Alcohol and Health: Current Evidence,* a bimonthly, free newsletter. Past articles have included "Safe Drinking Recommendations Should Vary by Age and Sex," "Reducing Mortality: Is Wine or Beer Better?," "Cognitive Effects of Moderate Alcohol Consumption," and more.

Alcohol and Your Health (Mayo Clinic)
<http://www.mayoclinic.com/invoke.cfm?id=SC00024>

The renowned Mayo Clinic has locations in Rochester, Minnesota; Jacksonville, Florida; and Scottsdale, Arizona. The Mayo Clinic's consumer health site includes information about the effects of alcohol on health, including the benefits of moderate alcohol consumption, and the side effects of excessive alcohol consumption.

Alcohol Use and Abuse
<http://www.niapublications.org/engagepages/alcohol.asp>

The National Institute on Aging's AgePage features information about alcohol abuse, the dangers of late onset problem drinking, sensitivity to alcohol in older drinkers, and symptoms of problem drinkers. The site content is available in English and Spanish languages.

Does Moderate Alcohol Use Prolong Life?
<http://www.acsh.org/healthissues/newsID.823/healthissue_detail.
  asp>

The American Council on Science and Health (ACSH) site features this article which discusses the potential for prolonging life through moderate alcohol consumption, as written by Dr. R. Curtis Ellison, professor of preventive medicine and public health at Boston University School of Medicine. The article discusses reduced risk of heart disease and death for moderate drinkers, and the dangers of excessive alcohol consumption.

Healthy Nutrition—The Effects of Alcohol
<http://www.anti-aging-guide.com/41alcohol.php>

This anti-aging guide was developed by Arcady L. Economo, who holds doctoral degrees (including one in pharmacy) and is associated with Anti-Aging Europe <http://www.antiaging-europe.com>. The guide's outline format includes abstracts from recent research articles on a variety of topics related to the subject. The research abstracts about the effects of alcohol include the healthy benefits of drinking wine, effects of alcohol on memory, the association of alcohol consumption with high-density lipoproteins, and more.

Resveratrol May Activate "Longevity Gene"
<http://www.mercola.com/2003/oct/1/longevity_gene.htm>

The aim of Dr. Joseph Mercola's site is to provide "comprehensive, clear and researched guidance on the best nutrition, medical, emotional therapy and lifestyle choices to improve and maintain total health." Resveratrol, an antioxidant that is found in the skin of grapes, is believed to have many health benefits from increasing longevity to preventing blood clots.

Women, Drinking, and Health
<http://www.indiana.edu/~engs/articles/women.html>

Professor Ruth C. Engs received permission from Harwood Press to post the text of her article about how women who drink moderately can prevent heart attack. Published in *Current Opinion in Psychiatry* in 1996, the article points out that many previous research studies have focused on alcohol consumption in males, and that moderate drinking in females has been associated with lower mortality, mostly due to a decrease in coronary heart disease.

ANTIOXIDANTS, VITAMINS, MINERALS, AND SUPPLEMENTS

☑ Antioxidants (MedlinePlus)
<http://www.nlm.nih.gov/medlineplus/antioxidants.html>

MedlinePlus is a consumer health resource developed by the U.S. National Library of Medicine that provides extensive information about more than 650 diseases and conditions. The information about antioxidants includes latest news, overviews, clinical trials, related issues (role of antioxidants in preventing cancer, for example), research, directory of nutrition professionals, and organizations.

Antioxidants (WebMD)
<http://my.webmd.com/hw/diet_and_nutrition/tp21273.asp>

WebMD includes useful content including diseases and conditions, symptoms, drugs and herbs, health and wellness, diet and nutrition, and more. Site information includes an overview of the use of dietary supplements including antioxidants to treat and prevent a wide range of serious diseases (cancer, macular degeneration, heart disease, Alzheimer's disease, arthritis, etc.).

Antioxidants and Health
<http://www.enzo.co.nz/antiox.html>

Enzo Nutraceuticals is a New Zealand–based company that processes pine bark to produce antioxidant capsules. The site's information discusses the health benefits of naturally produced and dietary supplement antioxidants, explains how oxygen free radicals cause oxidative stress and cell damage, lists the diseases associated with this damage, and the role that flavonoids play in preventing diseases, fighting age-related changes, and promoting good health.

Antioxidants: Your Modern Day Anti-Aging Nutrient
<http://www.fnri.dost.gov.ph/wp/antioxidants.htm>

The Department of Science and Technology (DOST) is mandated by the government of the Philippines "to provide central direction, leadership, and coordination of all science and technology activities in the country." DOST's Food and Nutrition Research Institute (FNRI) site includes information about food technologies, nutrition statistics, institute publications, and related links. The content about antioxidants explains how antioxidants neutralize the harmful effects of oxygen free radicals, recommends frequent consumption of various fruits and vegetables, and lists sources of natural oxidants.

Flavonoids and Carotenes
<http://www.anti-aging-guide.com/51flavonoids.php>

This anti-aging guide was developed by Arcady L. Economo, who holds doctoral degrees (including one in pharmacy) and is associated with Anti-Aging Europe <http://www.antiaging-europe.com>. The information about flavonoids includes research abstracts about flavonoid intake and the risks of different diseases (stroke, stomach cancer, etc.).

Flavonoids—The New Rage
<http://healthfullife.umdnj.edu/archives/new_rage_archive.htm>

The Healthful Life Project publishes a newsletter about living a healthier life and promotes a Health-Full-Life Program that recommends specific tests, comprehensive preventative physical examination, and a series of lifestyle changes that focus on good nutrition, weight control, regular exercise, and nonsmoking. The project's site includes information about flavonoids in grapes, wine, teas, vegetables, and fruits, and their reported health benefits.

Food Choice Pyramid
<http://www.drlam.com/pyramid.cfm>

Dr. Michael Lam is a physician who specializes in nutrition and anti-aging. The site's food pyramid recommends sweets and lean red meat once per week; free-range poultry and/or cold-water fish twice per week; and oil from olives, fish, or poultry, organic eggs, low-glycemic-index fruits, legumes, nuts, aboveground leafy green vegetables, low-glycemic-index whole grains every day. Dr. Lam also recommends drinking ten to twelve glasses of filtered water per day, and explains the types of foods that have a low glycemic index.

Maintaining Nutrition As We Age
<http://ohioline.osu.edu/ss-fact/0207.html>

The Ohio Department of Aging and Ohio State University Extension provide text and PDF versions of this information (written by a dietetic intern and nutrition specialist associated with Ohio State University). The major points include aging processes that may affect appetite and taste; the importance of fiber, calcium, vitamins A, B12, C, and D; and using the food guide pyramid (included as a color illustration) to make daily food choices.

☑ Nutrition and Aging: Vitamins and Minerals
<http://nirc.cas.psu.edu/pdf/Vit_min_overview.pdf>

The Pennsylvania State University Nutrition & Extension Partnership Project developed this nine-page document in 2001 to explain "vitamin and mineral needs of older adults, challenges in meeting those needs, and considerations for recommending a vitamin/mineral supplement." Information includes dietary reference intakes (DRIs) for adults aged fifty-one years and older, factors that affect micronutrient intake, nutrients that are essential for older adults, and more.

Phytochemicals
<http://food.oregonstate.edu/c.html>

Oregon State University's Food Source site includes this brief information about phytochemicals that act as antioxidants and the foods that contain these substances, links to other sites, and bibliographic citations related to the subject.

Phytochemicals (5 A Day the Color Way)
<http://www.5aday.com/html/consumers/scientists.php>

The 5 A Day the Color Way site promotes the daily consumption of five to nine colorful fruits and vegetables (see Figure 6.1). The site explains how phytochemicals help protect the body against cancer, the debilitating effects of aging, heart disease, vision loss, and more.

Phytochemicals: Guardians of Our Health
<http://www.andrews.edu/NUFS/phyto.html>

Dr. Winston J. Craig, professor of nutrition at Andrews University, a Seventh-day Adventist educational institution in Berrien Springs, Michigan, developed this continuing education information site about phytochemicals including the importance of eating fruits and vegetables, specific plants and foods that help protect against diseases such as cancer, and other health benefits of specific foods, herbs, and some food pigments.

Vitamins, Minerals, and Their Benefits
<http://www.watercress.co.uk/health/benefits.shtml>

This United Kingdom–based site about eating and preparing dishes made with watercress includes information written by dietitian Lyndel Costain about the health benefits of vitamins A, B1, B6, C, E, and K; minerals including calcium, iodine, iron, manganese, phosphorus, potassium, zinc, and magnesium; and phytochemicals.

☑ Vitamins and Minerals (MedlinePlus)
<http://www.nlm.nih.gov/medlineplus/vitaminsandminerals.html>

MedlinePlus is a consumer health resource developed by the U.S. National Library of Medicine that provides extensive information about more

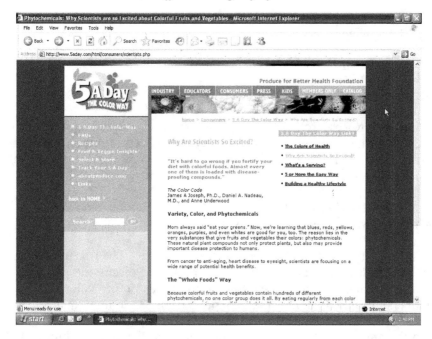

FIGURE 6.1. Phytochemicals
<http://www.5aday.com/html/consumers/scientists.php>
Used with permission.

than 650 diseases and conditions. The information about vitamins and minerals includes latest news; overviews; clinical trials; specific conditions (role of supplements in preventing heart disease, for example); prevention/screening; related issues; (role of antioxidants in preventing cancer); research; directory of nutrition professionals; supplements for children, teenagers, or seniors; and organizations.

DIET

Academy of Anti-Aging
<http://www.naturfood.net/eng/about.html>

The Israel Academy of Anti-Aging "is a society of potential long-livers created for exchange of experience and knowledge." Site information includes articles and book chapters about raw foods and immunity, links to sites about eating raw foods, and a Web-based forum for discussing raw and vegan diets.

The Anti-Aging Diet? Calorie Restriction: What is Calorie Restriction?
<http://www.anti-aging-research.us/p/163.html>

Anti-Aging-Research is a public information project sponsored by Medaus, a manufacturer of pharmacy solutions. The information about calorie restriction explains the practice, details how it may reduce cell damage, and discusses its effects on quality of life.

Calorie Restriction (CR) Society
<http://www.calorierestriction.org/>

This society's motto is "fewer calories, more life." The free basic membership entitles members to join the e-mail–based discussion list that includes information on the health benefits of restricting calories. Other memberships and donations range in price from $35 to more than $1,000. The information about calorie restriction (CR) includes video and slides from the annual conference, opportunities to participate in a human CR study, ways to "replace calorie-dense foods with calorie-sparse, nutrient-dense foods," recipes, potential risks and dangers, and links to external sites.

☑ Challenges and Choices: Fit for Life
<http://muextension.missouri.edu/xplor/hesguide/humanrel/gh6655.htm>

The University of Missouri Extension's Department of Food Science and Human Nutrition provides detailed information about eating more fruits, vegetables, and fiber; offers suggestions for each meal, cooking methods, and tips for eating out; suggests physical activities; and more. The information is available in HTML and PDF form.

The Importance of Low Glycemic Index in Anti-Aging
<http://www.anti-aging-guide.com/41glycemic.php>

This anti-aging guide was developed by Arcady L. Economo, who holds doctoral degrees (including one in pharmacy) and is associated with Anti-

Aging Europe <http://www.antiaging-europe.com>. The glycemic index information explains how different foods influence blood sugar levels, and includes research article citations and abstracts about how a low index can fight the effects of aging.

The Macrobiotic Guide
<http://www.macrobiotics.co.uk/>

Vitalise Wellbeing <http://www.Vwellbeing.com/>, a natural health care business, manages and updates this guide about eating whole grains, vegetables, and proteins derived from vegetable sources. Information includes the history of macrobiotics, dietary guidelines recipes, importance of chewing thoroughly, and the relationship of these practices to well-being and long life.

The Mediterranean Diet Pyramid
<http://www.oldwayspt.org/pyramids/med/p_med.html>

Oldways is a site that promotes "healthy eating, sustainable food choices, and traditional foodways," referring to the way that people in "olden times" ate. The diet pyramid features daily physical activity and consumption of olive oil, cheese, yogurt, whole grains, fruits, and vegetables; weekly consumption of eggs, fish, poultry, and sweets; and monthly consumption of red meats. This site also includes pyramids representing vegetarian, Asian, and Latin American diets (see Figure 6.2).

Omega-3 Fatty Acids: Are you Getting Enough? (MedicineNet.com)
<http://www.medicinenet.com/script/main/art.asp?articlekey=
41236>

Launched in 1996, MedicineNet.com features health content developed by over 70 U.S. board certified physicians. This information about the health benefits of fish oils quotes primary care physician Ann Gregorie Kulze, and nutrition expert Shawn Talbott, PhD. Sources of omega-3 fatty acids include salmon, sardines, herring, halibut, mackerel, bluefish, tuna, and other cold-water fish, as well as fish-oil supplements. Health benefits include preventing cancer, promoting weight loss, protecting the heart, controlling diabetes mellitus, and alleviating arthritis pain.

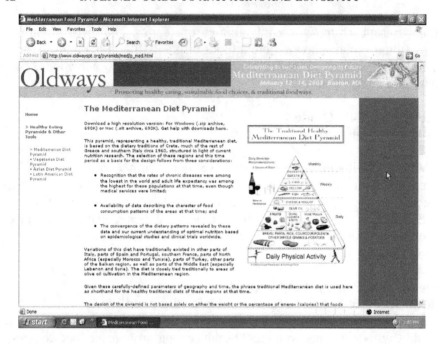

FIGURE 6.2. Mediterranean Diet Pyramid
<http://www.oldwayspt.org/pyramids/med/p_med.html>
Used with permission. Copyright 2000 Oldways Preservation & Exchange Trust.

Perricone Diet Review
<http://www.nvperriconemd.com/>

Nicholas V. Perricone is a Connecticut-based dermatologist who specializes in anti-aging treatments and dietary approaches, including his Three-Day Nutritional Face-lift and meal plan. The Perricone diet is characterized by the choice of carbohydrates with a low glycemic index; fresh or frozen fruits and vegetables; protein from fish (especially salmon), turkey, and chicken; nutritious dietary fats such as olive oil; selected dairy products; and water.

Raw Foodism
<http://www.vegetarianheadquarters.com/resource/Raw.htm>

The Vegetarian Headquarters site "is a resource tool that offers . . . the latest updates in news, articles, organizations and . . . more." The information about eating raw foods includes annotated links to external sites.

FITNESS REGIMENS

Exercise: The Ultimate Anti-Aging Pill
Study Finds That Both Weight and Exercise Are Key to Longevity
<http://www.hsph.harvard.edu/press/releases/press12222004.html>

This news item, from the Harvard School of Public Health, was released on December 22, 2004. It states that research findings appearing in the December 23, 2004, issue of *The New England Journal of Medicine* show that high body mass indices and decreased levels of physical activity were shown to contribute to "premature death in women."

Tai Chi for Longevity and Health
<http://www.mindbodypro.com/learningcenter/tai-chi.htm>

The International Association of Mind-Body Professionals (IAMBP) site explains the health benefits of tai chi, a physical activity that improves balance and strength, which can reduce the risk of falling and improve physical functions in older adults.

Walking for Health
<http://www.ramblers.org.uk/info/everyone/health.html>

The Ramblers' Association is a United Kingdom–based charity that has promoted walking for more than seventy years. The site includes information about the health benefits of walking including increased longevity, weight control, mental health, and more. *Take 30: A Practical Guide to Walking to Improve Health and Well Being* is (freely) downloadable from this site. A colorful poster titled *Take 30* detailing a ten-week plan to improve health through walking is available free upon request.

GENETICS AND HEREDITY

Anti-Aging Rx
<http://www.prevention.com/article/0,5778,s1-5-76-9-3691-1,00.html>

Rodale Press's *Prevention* magazine offers advice about fighting aging at "35, 45, 55, and beyond." Strategies relate to protecting the face from sun damage and strengthening the body at different stages in life.

Genes and Cancer
<http://www.biorap.org/br6rtoday.html>

Biological Research for Animals and People (BioRap) is an educational site that was developed by a coalition of educational institutions, health-related corporations, hospitals, and other organizations interested in aging and genetics, product safety, cancer, sun and skin, AIDS, risk assessment, and related information. The information about aging and genetics includes learning issues for students, lesson plans for teachers, and bibliographic citations related to the subject.

Genetics in Aging
<http://www.agingresearch.org/geneticsinaging/gtx_1_3.html>

This site is sponsored by the Alliance for Aging Research. Its motto is "Advancing Science, Enhancing Lives." The information about genetics explains gene testing, genes and disease, and understanding the results of genetic tests.

Genetics of Alzheimer's Disease
<http://www.healingwell.com/library/alzheimers/info2.asp>

HealingWell.com is a site that provides "health resources and interactive tools to enable patients to take control of their illness and start the healing process." These include resources on a wide range of health conditions which feature medical news, health articles, doctor-produced video Webcasts, message boards and chat rooms, e-mail, newsletters, books and reviews, and resource directories. The information about the genetics of Alzheimer's disease discusses the incomplete understanding of how genes cause disease, possible environmental factors, types of Alzheimer's disease (familial or sporadic), medical tests, genetic counseling, and avenues for future research.

Look & Feel Ten Years Younger
<http://www.prevention.com/article/0,5778,s1-1-93-9-323-1,00.html>

Rodale Press's *Prevention* magazine offers advice about ways to look and feel younger including exercising during pregnancy, starting resistance or strength training, maintaining good posture, exercising in the water, and more.

MARRIAGE OR COMMITTED RELATIONSHIPS

Grow Old Along with Me
<http://www.rand.org/publications/RB/RB5011/>

The RAND Corporation is a think tank that studies the "challenges facing the public and private sectors around the world." RAND's discussion of the health benefits of marriage covers research showing that "both men and women benefit from being married and both are at greater risk of dying, at any age, when they are not married—whether never married, separated, divorced, or widowed." The information is illustrated with a graph showing that "when marriage ends, only widowed women seem to retain some of the protective effects of marriage."

Married Adults Are Healthier
<http://www.worldhealth.net/p/248.html>

The American Academy of Anti-Aging Medicine (A4M), with more than 12,500 physicians and scientists as members, is a nonprofit, professional organization "dedicated to the advancement of technology to detect, prevent, and treat aging related disease and to promote research into methods to retard and optimize the human aging process." A4M's WorldHealth.net site includes information about aging theories, directories of anti-aging practitioners and clinics, an anti-aging glossary, research abstracts, clinical trials, and more. The information about health benefits derived from marriage refers to a study conducted by the U.S. Centers for Disease Control and Prevention (CDC).

Relationships Give Women Longevity
<http://www.hon.ch/News/HSN/514469.html>

The Health on the Net (HON) Foundation is an organization based in Switzerland that developed MedHunt, an English/French medical search engine, and a set of standards for evaluating sites with medical content. HON's news information about how women may benefit from relationships cites a study that was published in an issue of *Psychosomatic Medicine.*

MENTAL DISORDERS AND MENTAL HEALTH

Dementia Facts and Figures
<http://www.kingshill-research.org/whatis/facts.asp>

Kingshill Research Centre is part of the Department of Old Age Psychiatry (DOAP) and the Avon and Wiltshire Mental Health Partnership NHS Trust at Victoria Hospital in Swindon, Wiltshire, United Kingdom. The information about dementia includes prevalence of the disease in different age groups, number of people in the United Kingdom who have dementia, a percentage breakdown of the types of dementia (Alzheimer's disease, vascular dementia, dementia with Lewy bodies, fronto-temporal dementia, and others), and estimates of future dementia prevalence in the United Kingdom.

Elderly Mental Health
<http://www.mentalhealth.samhsa.gov/highlights/november2004/
alzheimers/topics.asp>

The Substance Abuse and Mental Health Services Administration (SAMHSA) of the U.S. Department of Health and Human Services (HHS) fields questions from the media, public, and health professionals about mental health. The SAMHSA site information about mental health in older persons includes Internet links, toll-free help lines for mental health information, information about Alzheimer's disease, and more.

Mental Health of the Elderly
<http://www.healthyminds.org/mentalhealthofelderly.cfm>

The American Psychiatric Association (APA) site explains that based on research, "elderly people are at greater risk of mental disorders and their complications than are younger people." Risks include depression, different types of dementia, disorientation or confusion unrelated to dementia, and Alzheimer's disease.

PET OWNERSHIP

Animals and Public Health
<http://www.achp.health.usyd.edu.au/pets/furber.html>

A symposium about animals and community health and public policy was held at the University of Sydney in 1998. This document reviews the effects of companion animals on the quality of life in older persons.

Benefits of Pet Ownership
<http://www.secondchanceforanimals.org/benefits_of_pet_ ownership.htm>

"Second Chance for Animals, Inc. is a not-for-profit volunteer group devoted to enhancing the lives, adoption rates, and experiences of the animals living in shelters." The organization's site lists some of pet ownership's health benefits including lower blood pressure, lower cholesterol levels, increased physical activity especially for dog owners, fewer doctor's visits required by elderly pet owners, and more.

☑ Health Benefits of Animals
<http://www.deltasociety.org/dsc000.htm>

The nonprofit Delta Society is an "international resource for the human-animal bond," that strives to improve "human health through service and therapy animals." Service animals assist persons with disabilities. Therapy animals interact with and visit persons who are ill, confined, and/or recovering. Site resources related to the health benefits of animal interactions include a bibliography, publications, calendar of events, and more.

Health Benefits of Pet Ownership Fact Sheet
<http://www.appma.org/press_industrytrends.asp>

The American Pet Products Manufacturers Association (APPMA) is a nonprofit organization whose mission "is to promote, develop and advance pet ownership and the pet product industry and to provide the services necessary to help its members prosper." The site briefly mentions studies that showed lower blood pressure levels, reduced stress, reduced heart disease, lower health care costs, and less loneliness and depression among pet owners.

Pets for the Elderly Foundation
<http://petsfortheelderly.org/Research.htm>

Pets for the Elderly Foundation is an Ohio-based nonprofit organization that "makes donations to animal shelters throughout the United States to enable them to provide elderly persons a companion pet at no charge." The site summarizes research about the health benefits of pet ownership for older adults including reducing risk of heart disease, improving mental health, power of pet therapy, and more.

☑ Physical & Medical Health Benefits
<http://www.peteducation.com/article.cfm?cls=0&cat=1491& articleid=638>

PetEducation.com is a "source for expert pet information," including drug information, alternative health care, veterinary procedures, clinic cases, first aid, and more, for a wide variety of animals including dogs, cats, fish, birds, ferrets, reptiles, and other small pets (gerbils, hamsters, rabbits, etc.). The information about the health benefits for humans who own pets includes increased longevity after heart attacks, lower cholesterol levels, reduced stress, lower blood pressure levels, increasing physical activity, decreased tremor and seizure activity, etc.

SEXUALITY AND SEXUAL DISORDERS

Aging and Human Sexuality Resource Guide
<http://www.apa.org/pi/aging/sexuality.html>

The American Psychological Association's guide to aging and sexuality includes a discussion about negative stereotypes about aging and sexuality; research article abstracts on sexual function in older adults, attitudes toward senior sexuality, sexual satisfaction in older adults, and more; annotated bibliography of books and multimedia; and links to external sites.

Aging Changes in the Female Reproductive System
<http://www.healthscout.com/ency/article/004016.htm>

HealthScout is a health portal that syndicates the use of health news, services, and tools for use on other sites. The information about age-related changes includes falling hormone levels, menopause, and common problems (uterine prolapse, pain during intercourse, vaginal dryness, osteoporosis).

Erectile Dysfunction (eMedicine)
<http://www.emedicine.com/med/topic3023.htm>

eMedicine is a site intended for health professionals that also includes useful consumer health information which requires free registration. The section about erectile dysfunction includes articles about the causes, diagnosis, and nonsurgical and surgical treatment of this condition, and related topics. Additional site information includes a medical dictionary, drug recalls and alerts, and useful tools for calculating ideal weight, body mass index, and more.

Erectile Dysfunction (MedicinePlus)
<http://www.nlm.nih.gov/medlineplus/erectiledysfunction.html>

MedlinePlus is a consumer health resource developed by the U.S. National Library of Medicine that provides extensive information about more than 650 diseases and conditions. The information about erectile dysfunction includes latest news, overviews, diagnosis/symptoms, treatment, clinical trials, alternative therapy, research, dictionary/glossaries, directories, organizations, statistics, and information specific to seniors.

Female Libido
<http://www.obgyn.net/infertility/infertility.asp?pages/news/ASRM-101102-12>

OBGYN.net is a site that focuses on "resources you might find at a medical conference or Women's Health symposium." This information was derived from findings presented by the University of Pennsylvania researchers at the 58th Annual Meeting of the American Society for Reproductive Medicine held in October 2002 in Seattle, Washington. The major point of the study is that low sexual desire relates to varying or fluctuating levels of testosterone in females rather than low levels.

Lifelong Sexuality
<http://www.helpguide.org/aging/sexuality_aging.htm>

Helpguide is "expert, non-commercial information on mental health and lifelong wellness: a project of the Rotary Club of Santa Monica and Center for Healthy Aging." The information about lifelong sexuality includes changes in men and women, medical conditions that can affect sexual interest and/or performance, safe sex, and links to other sources of information.

Myths of Aging
<http://www.psichi.org/pubs/articles/article_38.asp>

Psi Chi, the National Honor Society in Psychology, posted this special topic about the myths of aging. Written by Florence L. Denmark of Pace University, the site discusses some myths such as older adults being depressed, obsessed with youth, alienated by society, asexual, unattractive, etc. Denmark debunks these myths with research and statistics.

Physical Fitness, Aging, and Sexuality
<http://www.50plus.org/Libraryitems/3_6_Phys_Fit_aging_sexuality.html>

Fifty-Plus Lifelong Fitness, originated at Stanford University, is "a nonprofit organization whose mission is to promote an active lifestyle for older people." The organization site features information about fitness challenges, discussion group meetings in different states, news, articles, links to external sources of information, and more. The document about aging and sexuality discusses results of a survey administered to the organization's membership. Survey results "indicated a high level of sexual activity and satisfaction in both older men and women of the Fifty-Plus Fitness Association members," and showed a correlation between sexual satisfaction and "the degree of fitness."

SeniorSex.org: Older Adult Sex Reference
<http://instruct1.cit.cornell.edu/courses/psych431/student2000/dp51/external_links.html>

SeniorSex was developed by a Cornell University psychology student. Site features include information about ageism and sexuality, physiological changes, myths and facts about sexuality, sex tips, an online crossword that tests knowledge of sexuality in older persons, online attitude inventory, reviews of books about sex and aging, links to external resources, and more.

Sex After Sixty: A Natural Part of Life
<http://www.ncoa.org/content.cfm?sectionID=109&detail=134>

The National Council on Aging (NCOA) "is a national voice and powerful advocate for public policies, societal attitudes, and business practices that promote vital aging." The site features highlights of an NCOA study funded by Pfizer, Inc. that polled Americans over sixty about sexual activity, common sexual problems, talking to a physician about sexual issues, and more.

☑ Sex & Aging
<http://www.sexhealth.org/sexaging/>

Sexual Health infoCenter is a site that was developed originally by two University of Montreal students in 1997. The site includes several video clips and transcripts that feature several physicians discussing sex after age sixty, physical changes in men (primarily erectile dysfunction), physical changes in women (primarily vaginal dryness), and tips related to sexual stimulation, lubrication, and reducing stress.

Sex Over Sixty
<http://www.hc-sc.gc.ca/seniors-aines/naca/expression/15-2/exp15-2_1_e.htm>

Health Canada's Division of Aging and Seniors includes this information about sexuality later in life derived from a past issue of *Bulletin of the National Advisory Council on Aging*. Contents include discussions of normal aging processes; diseases, conditions, and medications that may affect sexual performance; lifestyle changes that can improve sexual desire and performance; health benefits of sexual activity; taboos and attitudes about sexual activity in later life; and a bibliography of books, journal articles, multimedia, and links to external sites.

Sexuality in Later Life
<http://www.niapublications.org/engagepages/sexuality.asp>

The U.S. National Institute on Aging's AgePage provides this information about sexual activity in older adults in both text and PDF formats. Points include normal physical changes, causes of sexual dysfunction, effects of surgery and drug therapy on sexual desire and function, safe sex, role of emotions in sexuality, and links to other sources of information.

SLEEP

Getting Your ZZZZZZZs: How Sleep Affects Health and Aging
<http://www.ilcusa.org/_lib/pdf/gettingzs.pdf>

International Longevity Center-USA (ILC-USA) is an affiliate of Mount Sinai's School of Medicine and functions as "a not-for-profit, nonpartisan research, policy and education organization whose mission is to help societies address the issues of population aging and longevity in positive and constructive ways." This nine-page document discusses the importance of getting enough sleep, including sleeplessness, snoring, sleep apnea, sleep deprivation, napping, relationship of exercise to sleep, tips for sleeping well, and more.

A Good Night's Sleep
<http://www.niapublications.org/engagepages/sleep.asp>

The National Institute on Aging's AgePage discusses the relationship between a good night's sleep and aging, common sleep problems such as insomnia and sleep apnea, ways to improve sleep habits, and additional resources. The content is available in English and Spanish languages.

Sleep
<http://www.worldhealth.net/p/281.html>

The American Academy of Anti-Aging Medicine, with more than 12,500 physicians and scientists as members, is a non-profit, professional organization "dedicated to the advancement of technology to detect, prevent, and treat aging related disease and to promote research into methods to retard and optimize the human aging process." A4M's WorldHealth.net site includes information about aging theories, directories of anti-aging practitioners and clinics, an anti-aging glossary, research abstracts, clinical trials, and more. The information about sleep discusses the relationship between sleep and increased death risk, sleep as a way to rescue memories, good sleep as a key to long life, and more.

Sleep, Health, and Aging
<http://www.ilcusa.org/_lib/pdf/ilcsleephealth1103.pdf>

International Longevity Center-USA (ILC-USA) is an affiliate of Mount Sinai's School of Medicine and functions as "a not-for-profit, nonpartisan research, policy and education organization whose mission is to help societies address the issues of population aging and longevity in positive and constructive ways." This thirty-six-page document discusses mechanisms of wakefulness and sleepiness; sleep disorders such as sleep apnea, sleep deprivation, insomnia, depression associated with insomnia, age-related changes in sleep patterns, menopause and sleep, memory and sleep, exercise and sleeping; napping in older persons; and future research directions.

Sound, Restful Sleep, and Anti-Aging
<http://www.immunesupport.com/bes038.htm>

Immune*Support*.com is a site that is sponsored and maintained by ProHealth, a company that conducts chronic fatigue syndrome and fibromyalgia research. The information about sleep is written by a physician and discusses how disruption of normal daytime and nighttime wake/sleep cycles can result in diseases, and how melatonin may help with these cycles, and fight the effects of aging.

Chapter 7

Experimental/Futuristic Approaches

CRYONICS AND CRYOGENICS

Alcor Life Extension Foundation
<http://www.alcor.org/>

Alcor used cryonic methods to preserve its first human body in 1976. The foundation site includes information about common myths about the subject, journal articles, publications, and more.

Cryonics Europe
<http://www.cryonics-europe.org/lr/lr86.htm>

"Cryonics Europe is a support and discussion group, based in Sussex, for people in Britain and the rest of Europe who are signed up for cryopreservation or who are considering it." Site features include information about preserving frozen bodies, technical issues, local events and meetings, and links to external sources of information.

Cryonics Institute Member Resources
<http://www.cryonics.org/info.html>

The Cryonics Institute "offers cryonic suspension services and information. As soon as possible after legal death, a member patient is prepared and cooled to a temperature where physical decay essentially stops, and is then maintained indefinitely in cryostasis. When and if future medical technology allows, our member patients hope to be healed and revived, and awaken to extended life in youthful good health." Site features include frequently asked questions, research updates and reports, membership information, release forms for cryonic suspension, links to external sources of information, and more.

The NanoAging Institute
<http://www.nanoaging.com/>

This institute concerns itself with life extension. The site's disclaimer states that site information is intended "to support, not replace, the relationship that exists between a patient/site visitor and his/her physician." Site features include a discussion forum; information about aging, centenarians, cloning, cryonics, diseases, longevity, oxidative damage, telomere, tissue engineering, transhumanism, etc.; news alerts; conferences; and more.

GENE THERAPY

Cancer: Gene Therapies, Stem Cells, Telomeres and Cytokines
<http://www.lef.org/protocols/prtcl-150.shtml>

Life Extension Foundation (LEF) "is a nonprofit organization, whose long-range goal is the radical extension of the healthy human lifespan." The foundation's site includes information about funded research, physicians who practice anti-aging medicine; eAdvisor, which details protocols about specific diseases and health concerns; specific anti-aging treatments including DHEA, human growth hormone, melatonin, and others; consumer alerts, news and a discussion forum; and services and products such as books, journal subscriptions, and anti-aging supplements. The site uses current research to explain how genes control cancer cells, the role of telomerase in cancer activity, stem cell transplants, and more.

Gene Manipulation
<http://www.anti-aging-guide.com/64gene.php>

This anti-aging guide was developed by Arcady L. Economo, who holds doctoral degrees (including one in pharmacy) and is associated with Anti-Aging Europe <http://www.antiaging-europe.com>. The information about gene manipulation includes research abstracts related to gene therapy for hemoglobin disorders and laboratory mice as animal models for determining whether oxidative stress causes aging.

Gene Therapy
<http://www.worldhealth.net/p/407.html>

The American Academy of Anti-Aging Medicine (A4M), with more than 12,500 physicians and scientists as members, is a nonprofit, professional organization "dedicated to the advancement of technology to detect, prevent, and treat aging related disease and to promote research into methods to retard and optimize the human aging process." A4M's WorldHealth.net site includes this information about gene therapy that reports on research related to repairing genetic damage in fruit flies, and gene therapy for a variety of diseases.

New Gene Therapy Fights Frailty
<http://www.sciencenews.org/pages/sn_arc98/12_19_98/fob1.htm>

Science News is published weekly and includes research developments in all fields of science. This article discusses loss of skeletal muscle due to aging, and how gene therapy may be useful in fighting associated frailty.

Targeted Genetics
<http://www.targen.com/basics/about-gt.php>

Targeted Genetics is a company that develops "molecular medicines to prevent or treat acquired, inherited and infectious diseases that have significant unmet medical need." The company's site includes information about gene therapy including basic information on the subject, clinical trials, glossary, and more.

HERBAL MEDICINE

American Herbal Pharmacopoeia (AHP)
<http://www.herbal-ahp.org/>

AHP's mission is "to promote the responsible use of herbal medicines" and ensure that "they are used with the highest degree of safety and efficacy as is achievable." Site features include press releases about published monographs, current news, ordering information for specific monographs, and more.

☑ Botanical.com
\<http://www.botanical.com/\>

Although this site functions primarily to sell herbal products, it also includes a message board and text of Maud Grieve's *A Modern Herbal,* which was published in 1931. Mrs. Grieve's book includes more than 800 varieties of herbs and plants, recipes, and a list of forty-four plants that are poisonous. For example, the information about Peruvian Bark includes a color image of the plant and its parts, synonyms, description, chemical constituents, medicinal actions and uses, and dosage. For instance, according to Grieve's work, fennel is said to convey longevity, and to give strength and courage.

☑ Herbal Medicine
\<http://www.nlm.nih.gov/medlineplus/herbalmedicine.html\>

MedlinePlus is a consumer health resource developed by the U.S. National Library of Medicine that provides extensive information about more than 650 diseases and conditions. The information about herbal medicine is not specific to anti-aging but includes latest news, overviews, pictures/diagrams, clinical trials, research, organizations, law and policy, and effects of herbs on women and children.

Herbal Remedies
\<http://www.all-natural.com/herbguid.html\>

The Natural Health and Longevity Resource Center site includes this guide about different herbal remedies. Although the information does not cite its sources, the annotated list ranges from alfafa (for treating fluid retention) to gotu kola ("longevity" herb) to yerba santa (for treating mucus in the respiratory tract).

Herbal Therapy and Elder Health
\<http://www.healthy.net/scr/article.asp?id=1919\>

HealthWorld Online is managed by a physician director and an advisory board of physicians, nurses, scientists, and other health professionals. The information about herbal therapy explains the psychology of aging, deriving most of the content from *Aging Well* by James F. Fries.

Herbs for Longevity
<http://www.findarticles.com/cf_dls/m0820/n234/19068904/p1/article. jhtml>

Originally printed in *Vegetarian Times* in 1997, this article by Luise Light explains how products of normal metabolism, such as oxygen free radicals, damage cells, tissues, and organs, and can lead to disease. FindArticles features more than 5 million articles from almost 1,000 sources, and is run by LookSmart, a search engine company.

Medherb.com
<http://www.medherb.com/>

The North American Institute of Medical Herbalism, Inc., publishes *Medical Herbalism,* and maintains this site that provides herbalism instruction, a free electronic herbalism newsletter, a threaded discussion board for reporting adverse effects of specific herbs, links to other information on the subject, and sells related publications.

HORMONE THERAPY

Can Hormones Prevent Aging?
<http://mdchoice.com/Pt/consumer/hormrev.asp>

MDchoice.com is a health and medicine portal that provides physician-reviewed content for consumer and health professionals in separate channels. This site's consumer channel is organized into centers including allergy, cancer, HIV and AIDS, children's health, diseases and medical conditions from acne to yellow fever, links to databases, and more. The information about hormones includes DHEA, human growth hormone, melatonin, testosterone, estrogen, and more.

Fibroblast Growth Factors
<http://www.drlam.com/A3R_brief_in_doc_format/fibroblast_ growth_factors.cfm>

Dr. Michael Lam is a physician who specializes in nutrition and anti-aging. Site information about fibroblast growth factors explains the different types, functions, and anti-aging effects.

Glucose, Hormones, Aging
<http://www.growyouthful.com/toc4horm.php>

The companion Web site to David Niven Miller's *Grow Youthful* includes an outline of information including this content about the relationship among glucose, hormones, and aging.

☑ **Growth Hormone: The Test**
<http://www.labtestsonline.org/understanding/analytes/growth_
    hormone/test.html>

Lab Tests Online is a peer-reviewed, noncommercial, patient-centered site that explains common laboratory tests and test results. The information about growth hormone explains how hormone levels are tested and why, and the significance of test results, factors that could affect test results, and other information.

☑ **Growth Hormone to Prevent Aging: Is It a Good Idea?**
<http://www.mayoclinic.com/invoke.cfm?id=HA00030>

The renowned Mayo Clinic has locations in Rochester, Minnesota; Jacksonville, Florida; and Scottsdale, Arizona, and maintains a number of Web sites of interest to health consumers. The information about growth hormone covers conventional uses of this substance to treat children with growth disorders, explains health benefits (increased bone density, increased body leanness, improved mood, etc.) for human growth hormone–deficient individuals, details side effects (fluid retention, heart failure, joint pain, hypertension, etc.), and calls for additional research.

Hormone Replacement
<http://www.worldhealth.net/p/264,5723.html>

The American Academy of Anti-Aging Medicine (A4M), with more than 12,500 physicians and scientists as members, is a nonprofit, professional organization "dedicated to the advancement of technology to detect, prevent, and treat aging related disease and to promote research into methods to retard and optimize the human aging process." A4M's WorldHealth.net site includes information about aging theories, directories of anti-aging practitioners and clinics, an anti-aging glossary, research abstracts, clinical trials, and more. The information about hormone therapy includes effects on the heart, brain, and risk of cancer.

☑ Hormone Replacement Therapy (MedlinePlus)
<http://www.nlm.nih.gov/medlineplus/hormonereplacementtherapy. html>

MedlinePlus is a consumer health resource developed by the U.S. National Library of Medicine that provides extensive information about more than 650 diseases and conditions. The information about hormone replacement therapy includes latest news, overviews, treatment, clinical trials, research, organizations, and more.

☑ Hormones (MedlinePlus)
<http://www.nlm.nih.gov/medlineplus/hormones.html>

MedlinePlus is a consumer health resource developed by the U.S. National Library of Medicine that provides extensive information about more than 650 diseases and conditions. The information about hormones includes overviews, anatomy/physiology, diagnosis/symptoms, treatment, research, directories, organizations, hormones as related to women, men, teenagers, and seniors, and more.

Human Growth Hormone
<http://www.worldhealth.net/p/349.html>

The American Academy of Anti-Aging Medicine (A4M), with more than 12,500 physicians and scientists as members, is a nonprofit, professional organization "dedicated to the advancement of technology to detect, prevent, and treat aging related disease and to promote research into methods to retard and optimize the human aging process." A4M's WorldHealth.net site includes information about aging theories, directories of anti-aging practitioners and clinics, an anti-aging glossary, research abstracts, clinical trials, and more. The information about human growth hormone describes its use to treat dwarfism and to alleviate age-related changes.

Testosterone
<http://www.worldhealth.net/p/4185.html>

The American Academy of Anti-Aging Medicine (A4M), with more than 12,500 physicians and scientists as members, is a nonprofit, professional organization "dedicated to the advancement of technology to detect, prevent, and treat aging related disease and to promote research into methods to retard and optimize the human aging process." A4M's WorldHealth.net site includes information about aging theories, directories of anti-aging practitioners and clinics, an anti-aging glossary, research abstracts, clinical trials, and more. The information about testosterone describes the hormone's major effects, signs and symptoms of low testosterone levels, testosterone replacement therapy, and related links.

TISSUE TRANSPLANTATION

Advances in Stem Cell Research
<http://www.worldhealth.net/p/416,1971.html>

The American Academy of Anti-Aging Medicine (A4M), with more than 12,500 physicians and scientists as members, is a nonprofit, professional organization "dedicated to the advancement of technology to detect, prevent, and treat aging related disease and to promote research into methods to retard and optimize the human aging process." A4M's WorldHealth.net site includes information about aging theories, directories of anti-aging practitioners and clinics, an anti-aging glossary, research abstracts, clinical trials, and more. The stem cell research information explains the usefulness of spleen stem cells, stem cell generation, U.S. federal and state government policy that threatens research, and more.

Artificial and Replacement Organs and Tissues
<http://www.worldhealth.net/p/393.html>

The American Academy of Anti-Aging Medicine (A4M), with more than 12,500 physicians and scientists as members, is a nonprofit, professional organization "dedicated to the advancement of technology to detect, prevent, and treat aging related disease and to promote research into methods to retard and optimize the human aging process." A4M's WorldHealth.net site includes information about aging theories, directories of anti-aging practitioners and clinics, an anti-aging glossary, research abstracts, clinical trials, and more. The information about organs and tissues includes information about the use of tissue engineering for blood vessels and knee cartilage, development of synthetic bone, and more.

Replacement Organs
<http://www.anti-aging-guide.com/65organs_PFV.htm>

This anti-aging guide was developed by Arcady L. Economo, who holds doctoral degrees (including one in pharmacy) and is associated with Anti-Aging Europe <http://www.antiaging-europe.com>. The information about replacement organs includes research abstracts about replacement hearts.

Stem Cell Therapy and Therapeutic Cloning
<http://www.anti-aging-guide.com/63stem.php>

This anti-aging guide was developed by Arcady L. Economo, who holds doctoral degrees (including one in pharmacy) and is associated with Anti-Aging Europe <http://www.antiaging-europe.com>. The information about stem cell therapy includes research abstracts about the potential use of human embryonic or adult stem cells in efforts to treat a wide range of diseases including spinal injuries, kidney disease, heart disease, diabetes mellitus, and others.

Stem Cells and Stem Cell Transplantation
<http://www.nlm.nih.gov/medlineplus/stemcellsandstemcell transplantation.html>

MedlinePlus is a consumer health resource developed by the U.S. National Library of Medicine that provides extensive information about more than 650 diseases and conditions. The information about stem cells includes latest news, overviews, treatment, clinical trials, directories, organizations, statistics, and minitransplants in seniors.

Chapter 8

Research

Centenarians
<http://www.hcoa.org/centenarians/centenarians.htm>

The Huffington Center on Aging (HCOA) at Baylor College of Medicine in Houston, Texas, focuses on many aspects of aging research including secretagogues, cognitive function, neurodegenerative diseases, tumor suppressor genes, and more. HCOA's information about centenarians includes examples of people who have lived longer than 100 years, including the late George Burns and the late Bob Hope.

Centenarians in the United States
<http://www.census.gov/prod/99pubs/p23-199.pdf>

Although this eighteen-page report was released by the U.S. Department of Health and Human Services in 1999, the work is based on the 1990 Census of Population and Housing. The information covers the cultural and scientific importance of studying centenarians, actual and projected statistics for the numbers of persons living to 100 and beyond, socioeconomic data, geographical distribution with most centenarians in 1990 living in California or New York, comparisons with centenarians living worldwide, and more.

Hutchinson-Gilford Progeria Syndrome
<http://www.ncbi.nlm.nih.gov/entrez/dispomim.cgi?id=176670>

Online Mendelian Inheritance in Man (OMIM) is a database that includes descriptions, citations, and genetic information about a wide array of diseases, medical conditions, and physiological processes. The information about precocious senility includes disease description, clinical features, genetics, and links to cited research.

Learning About Progeria
<http://www.genome.gov/11007255>

The National Human Genome Research Institute explains the relationship between heredity and progeria, a disease that is characterized by the rapid onset of aging in childhood. Progeria research has implications for future research into the physiology and prevention of aging processes.

☑ Longevity Genes: Hunting for the Secrets of the Centenarians
<http://www.ilcusa.org/_lib/pdf/longevitygenes5.04.pdf>

The International Longevity Center-USA (ILC-USA) is an affiliate of Mount Sinai's School of Medicine and functions as "a not-for-profit, non-partisan research, policy and education organization whose mission is to help societies address the issues of population aging and longevity in positive and constructive ways." This sixteen-page document covers the basics of genetics, explains the life spans of various animals, discusses how calorie restriction research has been shown to increase longevity, and elaborates on the quest for genes related to longevity. The document also includes a glossary and an annotated list of external sites with additional information.

The Longevity Genes Project
<http://www.aecom.yu.edu/home/longevitygenesproject/>

Albert Einstein College of Medicine at Yeshiva University in New York City is conducting a longevity genes project that is studying the genetic composition of Ashkenazi Jews. Ashkenazi Jews lived in eastern Europe (parts of Germany, Poland, and Russia). The project site includes frequently asked questions, preliminary results, research citations, news about the project in other publications, and more.

The New England Centenarian Study
<http://www.med.harvard.edu/programs/necs/centenarians.htm>

The New England Centenarian Study refers to a series of studies conducted by Harvard Medical School and Beth Israel Deaconess Medical Center. The Centenarian Prevalence Study "is an attempt to find and recruit all the centenarians (and their families) living in eight towns surrounding and including Boston, Massachusetts." As of December 31,

1996, the prevalence rate was determined to be about one centenarian per 10,000 people in this geographic area. The Population Genetics Study analyzes the pedigrees of these centenarians to determine the prevalence of longevity in families. The Extreme Longevity in Families Study "focuses on locating and verifying families with many members who have reached extreme age."

☑ The Okinawa Centenarian Study
<http://www.okinawaprogram.com/>

The Okinawa Centenarian Study is "a population-based study of hundred-year-olds (centenarians) and other elderly in Okinawa, Japan." The organization's site includes background information about the study, selection of research findings, video clips, position paper on coral calcium, news, and more.

Progeria
<http://www.rarediseases.org/search/rdbdetail_abstract.html?disname=
   Progeria%2C%20Hutchinson%20Gilford>

The National Organization for Rare Disorders (NORD) focuses on "orphan" diseases, or diseases that afflict fewer than 200,000 Americans. NORD's brief information about progeria includes an explanation of the disease and the gene mutations associated with it.

The Progeria Research Foundation Homepage
<http://www.progeriaresearch.org/>

Founded in 1999, the Progeria Research Foundation focuses on funding research projects related to treating and curing this disease, and offering resources and assistance to patients and their families. The foundation's site features information about diagnostic testing, patient registry, publications and research, health guidelines for families facing this disease, and more.

Progeria (Werner Syndrome)
<http://www.emedicine.com/derm/topic697.htm>

eMedicine is a site intended for health professionals that also includes useful consumer health information which requires free registration. The information about progeria includes pathophysiology, incidence, physical characteristics, and related diseases.

Research on Aging
<http://www.sri.com/policy/healthsci/aging/>

SRI International "is an independent, nonprofit research institute conducting contract research and development for government agencies, commercial businesses, foundations, and other organizations." SRI International was formerly known as Stanford Research Institute. Research at its Center for Health Sciences focuses on risk factors for death in aging adults and risk factors for premature aging of the brain. Site features include project descriptions, research abstracts, and links to external resources.

Werner Syndrome
<http://www.ncbi.nlm.nih.gov/entrez/dispomim.cgi?id=277700>

Online Mendelian Inheritance in Man (OMIM) is a database that includes descriptions, citations, and genetic information about a wide array of diseases, medical conditions, and physiological processes. The information about Werner syndrome, a group of physical signs and symptoms similar to progeria, includes clinical features, biochemical features, clinical management, genetic mutations, links to cited literature, and more.

Chapter 9

Interactive Tools

Every man desires to live long; but no man would be old.

Jonathan Swift

☑ AgeLine Database
<http://research.aarp.org/ageline/home.html>

The American Association of Retired Persons (AARP) is a nonprofit organization that focuses on issues and concerns of Americans who are fifty years of age and older. AgeLine indexes and abstracts geriatrics, gerontology, and aging-related research from other disciplines, including research journals, policy publications, consumer publications, academic dissertations, and more.

Anti-Aging Computer Tips
<http://www.aarp.org/computers-features/Articles/a2004-07-19-computertips>

The American Association of Retired Persons (AARP) is a nonprofit organization that focuses on issues and concerns of Americans who are fifty years of age and older. The AARP site suggests that solving a computer problem is an excellent way to keep the mind active and sharp, and contribute to lifelong learning. The information refers to tools on other sites that can help keep skills sharp.

Death Clock
<http://www.deathclock.com/>

This tool is a sobering visualization of how fleeting time can be on this earth depending on life expectancy and lifestyle habits. Based on answers to a number of questions (birth date, gender, temperament, body mass index, and smoking status), the clock estimates the number of seconds left, determines the likely date of a person's death, and links to the Life Extension Foundation site's top-ten listing of "nutrients, hormones, and drugs" believed to extend life.

Death Timer
<http://www.deathtimer.com/>

This site asks, "Do you know how much time you have left on this Earth?" This tool uses "published global life expectancy statistics to calculate . . . lifespan" based on answers to a few questions (birth date, country of residence, gender, smoker or nonsmoker, drinker of alcoholic beverages, overweight or not). The calculated, estimated death also lists the estimated death dates for the past five visitors to the site.

Eye Problems
<http://my.webmd.com/content/tools/1/slide_vision_test.htm?z=3628
    _81000_0000_09_01>

WebMD includes useful content about diseases and conditions, symptoms, drugs and herbs, health and wellness, diet and nutrition, interactive tools, and more. The information about eye problems adjusts an image to show how it looks to a person with macular degeneration, glaucoma, retinal detachment, floaters, cataracts, and color blindness compared to a person with normal vision.

Intelihealth Interactive Tools
<http://www.intelihealth.com>

Aetna, Inc., works with various partners (Harvard Medical School, University of Pennsylvania School of Dental Medicine) to provide access to consumer health content about diseases and conditions, healthy lifestyle, discussion boards, interactive tools, and more. The interactive tools include a body mass index calculator, depression self-assessment, heart and breath odometers, serving size surprise, and more.

☑ Live Well, Live Long
<http://www.asaging.org/cdc/>

This site's educational modules were developed by the American Society on Aging to promote healthy aging and include "Blueprint for Health Promotion," "Strategies for Cognitive Vitality," "Optimal Medication Use," "Road Map to Driving Wellness," "Mental Wellness," and more. These materials were "funded through a grant from the Centers for Disease Control and Prevention," and were "designed to increase understanding of the changing health and social service needs of an aging and more diverse population." The site requires free registration to access these materials.

Living to 100 Life Expectancy Calendar
<http://www.livingto100.com/>

This Web-based series of questions is intended to estimate life expectancy based on a number of factors including family history and lifestyle habits. In addition to receiving a numerical score, persons who complete the quiz are given feedback for each answer in an effort to encourage lifestyle changes that may benefit health and possible longevity.

Longevity
<http://www.ncbi.nlm.nih.gov/entrez/dispomim.cgi?id=152430>

Online Mendelian Inheritance in Man (OMIM) is a database that includes descriptions, citations, and genetic information about a wide array of diseases, medical conditions, and physiological processes. The information about longevity describes research studies about nonagenarians, Danish twins, animal models for long life, and more.

Longevity Game
<http://www.nmfn.com/tn/learner-life-events-longevity>

Northwestern Mutual Financial Network's game uses thought-provoking questions (age, gender, blood pressure measurement, family history of disease, smoking, drinking, driving, etc.) to calculate longevity.

Longevity Quiz
<http://www.thelivingcentury.com/pdf/longevity_quiz.pdf>

The Living Century is "a long-term public arts project that includes an award-winning PBS television series." The project's site includes this twenty-question quiz that can be scored to estimate life span. The quiz was developed by researchers at Harvard Medical School, based on a study of 150 centenarians.

One-Minute Osteoporosis Risk Test
<http://www.osteofound.org/osteoporosis/risk_test.html>

The Osteoporosis Foundation offers print and interactive versions of their osteoporosis risk test. The test features nine questions for women and eight questions for men. Test results advise whether an individual is at risk for developing the disease and whether one should consult a physician. This risk test is available in many languages including English, French, German, Italian, Portuguese, Spanish, Turkish, and others. The site also includes information about prevention, diagnosis, and treatment of this debilitating disease.

Online Checkups
<http://www.healthfinder.gov>

The National Health Information Center of the U.S. Department of Health and Human Services maintains Healthfinder as a source of authoritative health information. The online checkups on this site include tests of calcium knowledge, hydration, and more.

☑ Online Mendelian Inheritance in Man
<http://www.ncbi.nlm.nih.gov/entrez/query.fcgi?db=OMIM>

Online Mendelian Inheritance in Man (OMIM) is a database that includes descriptions, citations, and genetic information about a wide array of diseases, medical conditions, and physiological processes that have a genetic basis.

Public Health and Aging E-mail Forum
<http://www.cdc.gov/aging/forum.htm>

The U.S. Centers for Disease Control and Prevention (CDC) hosts an e-mail–based discussion group for persons interested in public health and aging.

☑ RealAge Test
<http://www.realage.com/>

RealAge's premise is that is it possible to look younger and live longer by paying attention to family history, diet, exercise, existing health conditions, personal habits, and other factors. The Web-based test features a long series of questions to determine biological age, and formulate a personalized plan. The site requires free registration to save data within the system.

Test Yourself!
<http://www.healthandage.com/Home/gm=4>

Health and Age's motto is "live well, live longer" and is "sponsored by the Web-based Health Education Foundation (WHEF), an independent non-profit organization," although the site was created originally "by the Novartis Foundation for Gerontology in 1998." Tests and tools include likelihood of having a heart attack, RiskFactor Roulette, body mass index calculator, test for depression in older people, sleep deprivation, and more.

ThirdAge—Games & Jokes
<http://www.thirdage.com/living/games/quizzes/>

This site is intended for persons in their thirties, forties, and fifties who are interested in personal growth and development. Jokes and games related to aging include Interactive Leonardo, Your Changing Body Quiz, Menopause Myths, and more.

What's Your Eye-Q
<http://agingeye.com/about/eye-q.php?VI=FALSE>

This site has a disclaimer that its content is intended for Canadian residents only. The site's editor in chief is a medical doctor. Two versions of the site content are presented: one with enlarged text and simplified design for visually impaired users, and the other with "standard form" for text size and site design, but the font size can be increased at any time. Eye-Q is a "quick test to find out if you are among the millions of older Americans who may have a vision problem and may benefit from an examination by an optometrist or ophthalmologist."

Chapter 10

Institutes, Clinics, Organizations, and Societies

Active Living Coalition for Older Adults (ALCOA)
<http://www.alcoa.ca/>

ALCOA is "a partnership of organizations and individuals having interest in the field of aging, encourages older Canadians to maintain and enhance their well-being and independence through a lifestyle that embraces daily physical activities." Site features include updates on various active living projects, research updates, e-mail–based discussion groups, links to external sites, and more. The content is available in English and French languages.

Administration on Aging (AoA)
<http://www.aoa.gov/>

AoA is an agency within the U.S. Department of Health and Human Services that focuses on promoting "the dignity and independence of older people" and helping "society prepare for an aging population." The AoA site includes content in Chinese, German, Korean, Spanish, French, Italian, Japanese, Portuguese, and English languages. Site features include news about aging, agency publications, publications from other government agencies, events, and more.

Age Concern England
<http://www.ace.org.uk/>

Age Concern is a United Kingdom–based organization that was formerly called National Old People's Welfare Committee. Site features include a discussion board, news, and links to external resources.

Alliance for Aging Research
<http://www.agingresearch.org/>

The Alliance for Aging Research's motto is "Advancing science. Enhancing lives." Site information includes research, health topics, publications, newsletter, resources, events, and links to external resources.

American Academy of Anti-Aging Medicine (A4M)
<http://www.worldhealth.net/>

A4M, with more than 12,500 physicians and scientists as members, is a nonprofit, professional organization "dedicated to the advancement of technology to detect, prevent, and treat aging related disease and to promote research into methods to retard and optimize the human aging process." A4M's WorldHealth.net site includes information about aging theories, directories of anti-aging practitioners and clinics, an anti-aging glossary, research abstracts, clinical trials, and more.

American Council on Science and Health (ACSH)
<http://www.acsh.org/>

ACSH is "a consumer education consortium concerned with issues related to food, nutrition, chemicals, pharmaceuticals, lifestyle, the environment and health. ACSH is an independent, nonprofit, tax-exempt organization." Site features include health issues (diseases, food safety, nutrition/lifestyle, etc.), news and commentary, publications including *Resolve to Be Healthy in 2005,* events (dinners, conferences, symposia, etc.), and facts and fears about issues related to science and health.

☑ American Federation for Aging Research (AFAR)
<http://www.afar.org/>

Established in 1981, AFAR's mission is "to promote healthier aging through biomedical research." Site features include news stories, publications (federation newsletter, annual report), and links to external government agencies and organizations related to aging. Other publications can be requested free of charge, and will be mailed, including *Lifelong:* Research News on Dementia; *Lifelong:* Research News on Older Men's Health; *Lifelong:* Research News on Older Women's Health; *Lifelong:* Biology of Aging: Caloric Restriction; *Lifelong:* Biology of Aging: Oxidative Damage; *Lifelong:* Biology of Aging: Telomeres, and others.

American Geriatrics Society (AGS)
<http://www.americangeriatrics.org/>

AGS is an organization of health professionals who are "dedicated to improving the health and well-being of all older adults." Site features include press releases, newsletters, facts and figures, clinical practice guidelines, position statements, information about trends in geriatrics training, and more.

American Society on Aging
<http://www.asaging.org/>

The American Society on Aging focuses on "enhancing the knowledge and skills of those working with older adults." Membership benefits include subscriptions to *Aging Today, ASA Connection,* and a choice of special focus groups. Nonmembers can access portions of these publications through the society's site.

AntiAging-Europe.com
<http://www.antiaging-europe.com/>

This organization is devoted to health promotion and life extension. Site features include current and archived news; information about obesity, psoriasis, cancer, colds and influenza, impotence, prostatic hyperplasia, and other medical conditions; and more.

Kronos Longevity Research Institute
<http://www.kronosinstitute.org/>

This institute claims to "focus on overall effects of aging, rather than disease cures." Current research projects include the effects of testosterone on arteriosclerosis in men, relationship of early hormone replacement therapy on arteriosclerosis, and progression of heart disease in persons with diabetes. Previous studies examined cancer detection, oxidative stress, and beneficial effects of foods containing omega-3 fatty acids.

☑ The Life Extension Foundation
<http://www.lef.org/anti-aging>

Life Extension Foundation (LEF) "is a nonprofit organization, whose long-range goal is the radical extension of the healthy human lifespan." The foundation's site includes information about funded research, physicians who practice anti-aging medicine; eAdvisor, which details protocols about specific diseases and health concerns; specific anti-aging treatments including DHEA, human growth hormone, melatonin, and others; consumer alerts, news, and a discussion forum; and products and services such as books, journal subscriptions, and anti-aging supplements (see Figure 10.1).

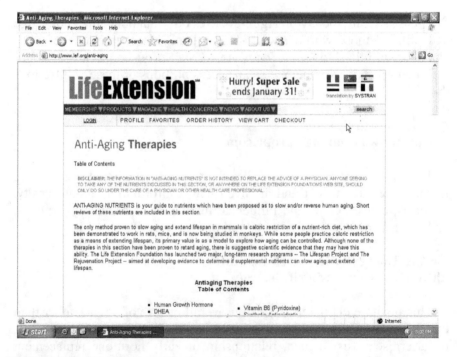

FIGURE 10.1. The Life Extension Foundation
<http://www.lef.org/anti-aging>
Used with permission.

Life Span Institute at the University of Kansas
<http://www.lsi.ku.edu/lsi/>

The Schiefelbush Institute for Life Span Studies at the University of Kansas "brings together scientists of diverse disciplines including psychology, psychiatry, speech pathology, sociology, education, biology, pharmacology, physiology and medicine to study human development from its genetic origins through the final stages of life." The site includes an overview of the institute's work including research being conducted at affiliated centers in Kansas and other states, directory of institute faculty and staff, state and regional services, current and past research projects, and a schedule of presentations given by affiliated researchers.

☑ The Merck Institute of Aging & Health
<http://www.merck.com/healthinfo/aging/1500.html>

Merck and Co., Inc., established Merck Institute of Aging & Health as "a nonprofit organization dedicated to improving the health and supporting the independence of older people around the world by communicating health information, educating the public and health professionals, and encouraging research in the field of health and aging." The institute site links to its aging and health site, *The Merck Manual of Health & Aging, The Merck Manual of Geriatrics,* and other useful information (see Figure 10.2).

The NanoAging Institute
<http://www.nanoaging.com/>

This institute concerns itself with life extension. The site's disclaimer states that site information is intended "to support, not replace, the relationship that exists between a patient/site visitor and his/her physician." Site features include a discussion forum; information about aging, centenarians, cloning, cryonics, diseases, longevity, oxidative damage, telomere, tissue engineering, transhumanism, etc.; news alerts; conferences; and more.

National Institute on Aging (NIA)
<http://www.nih.gov/nia/>

NIA is a U.S. government agency that "leads a broad scientific effort to understand the nature of aging and to extend the healthy, active years of

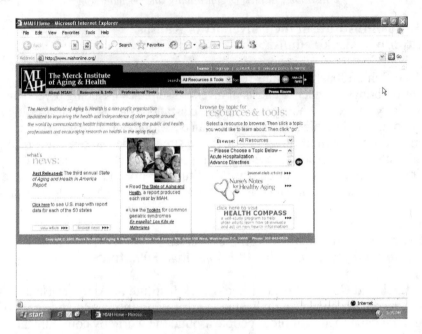

FIGURE 10.2. The Merck Institute of Aging & Health
<http://www.merck.com/healthinfo/aging/1500.html>
Used with permission.

life." Site features include publications, information about Alzheimer's disease, clinical trials that seek older research subjects, database of longitudinal studies, news and events, and links to other government sources of information.

State and Area Agencies on Aging
<http://www.aoa.gov/eldfam/How_To_Find/Agencies/Agencies.asp>

AoA is an agency within the U.S. Department of Health and Human Services that focuses on promoting "the dignity and independence of older people," and helping "society prepare for an aging population."

Strategies for Engineered Negligible Senescence (SENS)
<http://www.gen.cam.ac.uk/sens/>

As developed and maintained by biogerontologist Aubrey De Grey, associated with the Department of Genetics at the University of Cambridge in the United Kingdom, this unconventional site focuses on the application of "engineering principles to curing aging (reversing aging), not just slowing aging." The term "engineered negligible senescence" means creating a population that does not show signs of aging. Site features include links to *Rejuvenation Research,* published by Mary Ann Liebert, Inc.; answers to provocative questions such as how long a person can expect to live; conferences; and similar views written by others.

UCLA Center on Aging
<http://www.aging.ucla.edu/>

The UCLA Center on Aging's mission is "to enhance and extend productive and healthy life through preeminent research and education on aging." Site features include information about education, events, research, publications, and multimedia files of lectures about memory.

World Future Society (WFS)
<http://www.wfs.org/>

WFS is a nonprofit educational and scientific organization that was founded in 1966. The organization's site includes interviews with futurists, Web-based forums, publications, meetings, and information such as forecasts for the future, and more.

Chapter 11

Publications

☑ **Aging Begins at 30**
<http://www.vh.org/adult/patient/internalmedicine/aba30/>

The Virtual Hospital site provides access to Dr. Ian Maclean Smith's medical advice column dating back to 1992. The column appears weekly in *Iowa City Press Citizen*. Dr. Smith is professor emeritus at University of Iowa Hospitals and Clinics. Column topics are organized by year, medical discipline or organ system, and alphabetically by categories ranging from addictions to wellness. The columns have been peer reviewed internally, and represent sound health information on a wide range of topics for patients.

Aging & Its Implications: An Online Primer for Healthcare
    Professionals and Carers
<http://www.healthandage.com/html/res/primer/index.htm>

Health and Age's motto is "live well, live longer" and "is sponsored by the Web-based Health Education Foundation (WHEF), an independent non-profit organization," although the site was created originally "by the Novartis Foundation for Gerontology in 1998." This resource covers topics such as memory and mind; skin; heart and circulation; respiration; digestive system; eyes and ears; urinary system; muscles, bones, and joints; hormones and metabolism; and more.

The Aging Factor in Health and Disease: The Promise of Basic
    Research on Aging
<http://www.ilcusa.org/_lib/pdf/agingfactor.pdf>

International Longevity Center-USA (ILC-USA) is an affiliate of Mount Sinai's School of Medicine and functions as "a not-for-profit, nonpartisan research, policy and education organization whose mission is to help societies address the issues of population aging and longevity in positive and constructive ways." This twenty-six-page document was produced in conjunction with a workshop held in 1999, and details specific genes that have been shown to affect life spans in animal and organism models, future areas of research (biomarkers), glossary, and a list of citations.

Aging Today
<http://www.asaging.org/at/at.html>

The American Society on Aging publishes this newspaper every two months as a benefit to society members, or by subscription. Parts of each issue are available free to nonsubscribers through this site, which focuses on "public policy, research, practice, media and programming in the field of aging."

Alcohol and Health: Current Evidence
<http://www.bu.edu/act/alcoholandhealth/index.html>

Boston University publishes *Alcohol and Health: Current Evidence* as a free newsletter every two months. Past articles have included "Safe Drinking Recommendations Should Vary by Age and Sex," "Reducing Mortality: Is Wine or Beer Better?," "Cognitive Effects of Moderate Alcohol Consumption," and more.

Anti-Aging Newsletter
<http://www.anti-aging-newsletter.com/>

This free resource requires one-time registration. It offers "anti-aging therapies, including: diet, vitamins, hormone replacement therapy, advanced anti-aging products, exercise, stress reduction and much more."

☑ Biotech E-Newsletter
<http://www.worldhealth.net/p/642,6142.html>

The American Academy of Anti-Aging Medicine (A4M), with more than 12,500 physicians and scientists as members, is a nonprofit, professional organization "dedicated to the advancement of technology to detect, prevent, and treat aging related disease and to promote research into methods to retard and optimize the human aging process." This site includes articles derived from the literature such as how hot tea can prevent Alzheimer's disease, enlarged brain blood vessels may cause mental decline, why aging cells may be susceptible to cancer, and more.

Evolutionary Theories of Aging and Longevity
<http://www.longevity-science.org/Evolution.htm>

This article was originally published in *The ScientificWorldJOURNAL* and written by Leonid A. Gavrilov and Natalia S. Gavrilova of the Center on Aging at the University of Chicago. The authors discuss three evolutionary theories of aging including programmed death, mutation accumulation, and antagonistic pleiotropy.

☑ *Generations: Journal of the American Society on Aging*
<http://www.generationsjournal.org/>

The American Society on Aging publishes *Generations* as a means to disseminate information about aging to professionals in the field, and describes its audience as "administrators and managers, direct service providers, health and social services professionals, educators, researchers, students, policy makers and planners in all settings serving older adults and their families." Past articles have discussed hunger and aging, mobility, sensory impairment, and related topics. Nonsubscribers can access parts of current and past issues.

Geriatric Times
<http://www.geriatrictimes.com/>

Geriatric Times published "special reports, compelling editorial content, timely news coverage, continuing education articles, patient teaching aids and more." Although this publication ceased in November/December 2004, typical articles covered topics such as at-risk drinking in the older population, treatments for late-life depression, anti-aging elixirs, and more.

Health and Age Newsletters
<http://www.healthandage.com/Home/gm=22>

Health and Age's motto is "live well, live longer" and "is sponsored by the Web-based Health Education Foundation (WHEF), an independent non-profit organization," although the site was created originally "by the Novartis Foundation for Gerontology in 1998."

☑ Infoaging Publications
<http://www.infoaging.org/subscribe.html>

The American Federation for Aging Research (AFAR) developed this site with funding from Pfizer Inc. The site focuses on three major areas: biology of aging, disease center, and healthy aging. Publications can be requested through a Web-based form; topics include telomeres, oxidative damage, calorie restriction, and more.

International Longevity Center: Books and Reports
<http://www.ilcusa.org/pub/books.htm>

International Longevity Center-USA (ILC-USA) is an affiliate of Mount Sinai's School of Medicine and functions as "a not-for-profit, nonpartisan research, policy and education organization whose mission is to help societies address the issues of population aging and longevity in positive and constructive ways." This site includes publications about redesigning health care to serve older populations, longevity genes, the relationship between sleep and aging, use of testosterone to treat male menopause, biomarkers of aging, maintaining cognitive vitality, and more.

☑ *The Merck Manual of Health & Aging*
<http://www.merck.com/pubs/mmanual_ha/contents.html>

Merck and Company, Inc., publishes a number of useful reference works including portions of *The Merck Manual of Health & Aging*. Topics include "Fundamentals of Aging," "Caring for Self and Others," "Medical Conditions," "Social, Legal, and Ethical Issues," and essays about getting older, staying youthful, achieving one's dreams, and more (see Figure 11.1).

Older Americans 2004: Key Indicators of Well-Being
<http://www.agingstats.gov/default.htm>

The Federal Interagency Forum on Aging Related Statistics (AgingStats. Gov) provides free access to this 160-page publication that "covers 37 key indicators selected by the Forum to portray aspects of the lives of older

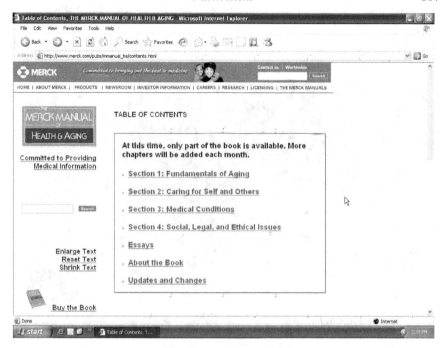

FIGURE 11.1. *The Merck Manual of Health & Aging*
<http://www.merck.com/pubs/mmanual_ha/contents.html>
From *The Merck Manual of Health & Aging,* edited by Mark H. Beers. Copyright 2004
by Merck & Co., Inc., Whitehouse Station, NJ.

Americans and their families. It is divided into five subject areas: population, economics, health status, health risks and behaviors, and health care."

Pocket Guide to Staying Healthy at 50+
<http://www.ahrq.gov/ppip/50plus/50plus.pdf>

The Agency for Healthcare Research and Quality (AHRQ), a division of the U.S. Department of Health and Human Services published this seventy-page guide in November 2003. Chapter topics include talking with physicians and nurses; lifestyle habits that reduce disease risks; health checkups and medical tests; seeking health information by telephone or online; and forms for tracking medical tests and checkups (see Figure 11.2).

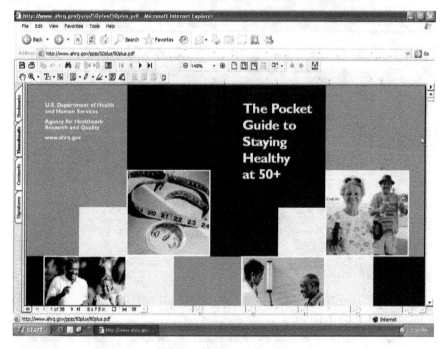

FIGURE 11.2. Pocket Guide to Staying Healthy at 50+
<http://www.ahrq.gov/ppip/50plus/50plus.pdf>

A Profile of Older Americans: 2002
<http://www.aoa.gov/prof/Statistics/profile/profiles2002.asp>

The Administration on Aging (AoA) is an agency within the U.S. Department of Health and Human Services that focuses on promoting "the dignity and independence of older people," and helping "society prepare for an aging population." This sixteen-page document details projected growth of the numbers of persons aged sixty-five and older through 2030; and marital status, racial and ethnic composition, geographic distribution, socioeconomic features, and more for older persons in the United States.

Rejuvenation Research
<http://www.liebertpub.com/publication.aspx?pub_id=127>

Mary Ann Liebert, Inc., publishes a number of scholarly journals including this one. Nonsubscribers can view tables of contents and some full-text content. *Rejuvenation Research* publishes research related to reju-venation therapies as well as "sociopolitical and ethical issues relating to substantial extension of healthy human life." Recent articles include "It's Never Too Late: Calorie Restriction Is Effective in Older Mammals," and "Table of World-Wide Living Supercentenarians for the Year 2003."

☑ *The State of Aging and Health in America 2004*
<http://www.cdc.gov/aging/pdf/State_of_Aging_and_Health_in_America_2004.pdf>

The U.S. Centers for Disease Control and Prevention (CDC) developed this forty-eight page report in conjunction with the Merck Institute of Aging & Health (see Figure 11.3). This third-annual publication provides a state-by-state report card on healthy aging, physical activity and older Americans, and gives examples from specific states such as Washington, Maine, North Carolina, and Kansas.

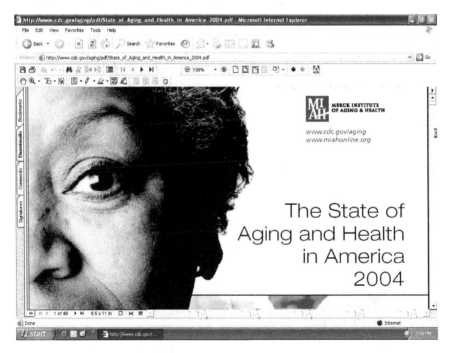

FIGURE 11.3. *The State of Aging and Health in America 2004*
<http://www.cdc.gov/aging/pdf/State_of_Aging_and_Health_in_America_2004.pdf>

Chapter 12

Statistics

Age Data
<http://www.census.gov/population/www/socdemo/age.html>

The U.S. Census Bureau organizes age adapt data from a number of sources: census data, estimates since the last census, annual topical surveys, and population projections. The data are available on the national level, by state, and by county. The Census Bureau also "conducts demographic and socioeconomic studies and strengthens statistical development around the world through technical assistance, training, and software products." The site also features reports and detailed tables for older (fifty-five years of age and older) and elderly (sixty-five years of age and older) populations.

☑ **AgingStats.Gov**
<http://www.agingstats.gov/>

Twelve U.S. federal agencies work together to collect and disseminate "data on the aging population." Useful site features include *Older Americans 2004: Key Indicators of Well-Being,* links to statistical sources, agency contacts, and more (see Figure 12.1).

Alliance for Aging Research
<http://www.agingresearch.org/aging_stats.cfm>

The Alliance for Aging Research's motto is "Advancing Science. Enhancing Lives." The site's useful statistical information includes the number of American medical schools that require geriatric training as part of the curriculum, incidence of age-related diseases in the population, number of Americans over age sixty-five, and more.

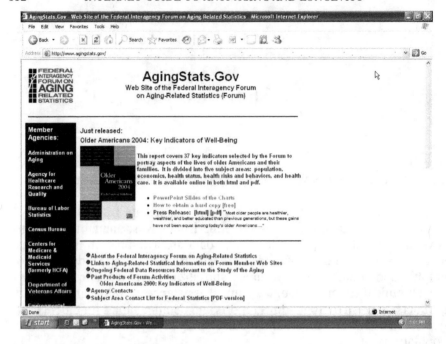

FIGURE 12.1. AgingStats.Gov
<http://www.agingstats.gov/>

Center on Population Health and Aging
<http://www.pop.psu.edu/cpha/resources.htm>

The mission of the Pennsylvania State University's Center on Population Health and Aging "is to provide a synergistic research environment supporting the development of innovative interdisciplinary research dealing with the challenges of a growing and increasingly diverse older population." Site features include links to aging centers funded by the National Institute on Aging, national and international organizations devoted to aging, and more.

Healthy Life Expectancy
<http://www3.who.int/whosis/hale/hale.cfm?path=whosis,burden_statistics,hale&language=english>

The World Health Organization Statistical Information Service (WHOSIS) provides "healthy life expectancy (HALE) . . . based on life expectancy

(LEX), but includes an adjustment for time spent in poor health" for persons residing in member states from Afghanistan to Zimbabwe.

Longevity
<http://www.worldhealth.net/p/267,6131.html>

The American Academy of Anti-Aging Medicine (A4M), with more than 12,500 physicians and scientists as members, is a non-profit, professional organization "dedicated to the advancement of technology to detect, prevent, and treat aging related disease and to promote research into methods to retard and optimize the human aging process." A4M's WorldHealth.net site includes information about aging theories, directories of anti-aging practitioners and clinics, an anti-aging glossary, research abstracts, clinical trials, and more. The information specific to longevity includes life extension statistics, centenarian statistics, longevity research, and articles related to extreme longevity.

Longevity Statistics—New Zealand
<http://www.stats.govt.nz/popn-monitor/longevity-new-zealanders/>

Statistics New Zealand (or Tatauranga Aotearoa in the Maori language) "is a government department and New Zealand's national statistical office." The information about longevity among New Zealanders includes a population clock, life expectancy at birth for the most recent period of time, and other graphs and tables that compare longevity for Maori and non-Maori persons living in New Zealand.

Statistics Canada
<http://www.statcan.ca/start.html>

The Canadian government's official statistics site "produces statistics that help Canadians better understand their country—its population, resources, economy, society and culture." Site features include census data, population maps, community profiles, publications, and links to external sites. Content is available in English and French languages.

Trends in Health and Aging
<http://www.cdc.gov/nchs/agingact.htm>

The U.S. Centers for Disease Control and Prevention (CDC) site offers information about aging links to the National Center for Health Statistics (NCHS) data including Trends in Health and Aging, Longitudinal Studies of Aging, and more.

Glossary

Some of the terms used throughout this guide may be unfamiliar to the layperson. These definitions and information about acronyms were derived from several excellent sources, including:

- **Medical Dictionary**
  <http://www.medical-dictionary.com/>
- **MedlinePlus Merriam-Webster Medical Dictionary**
  <http://www.nlm.nih.gov/medlineplus/mplusdictionary.html>
- **Skeptic's Dictionary**
  <http://skepdic.com/>

aboriginal: Native.

abstracts: Brief summaries of the major points of an article or research presentation.

acetyl-L-carnitine: A naturally occurring substance that helps the body develop muscle tissue, reduce body fat, and improve overall health.

acronyms: Words formed from the first letter or letters of words in a name or phrase, such as CDC for Centers for Disease Control and Prevention.

adult stem cells: *See* STEM CELLS.

aggregated: Collected or combined. Related to consumer health information, this term is used to indicate grouped resources that can be searched with a common interface.

allopathic medicine: Mainstream or conventional methods of diagnosing and treating diseases and health conditions. *See also* NATUROPATHIC MEDICINE.

alopecia: Hair loss.

andropause: Male MENOPAUSE, or age-related low levels of TESTOSTERONE.

annotated: With explanatory notes.

anthocyanins: Red or blue plant pigments believed to have health benefits.

antibodies: Proteins that protect against harmful substances such as bacteria or viruses.

antigens: Naturally occurring and introduced substances that stimulate an immune response.

antioxidants: Substances that slow the aging process and prevent disease; examples include vitamin E, beta-carotene, and BHT (butylated hydroxytoluene). Cereal manufacturers, for example, use BHT to coat cereal boxes to help keep the products fresh. *See also* OXYGEN FREE RADICALS.

assays: Analyses of substances to determine presence, absence, or quantity of one or more ingredients or parts. *See also* IMMUNOASSAYS.

authoritative: As related to Web site content, accurate and reliable.

bibliographic: As related to informational databases or reference lists, citations that include author, title, source, and abstract, elements that are needed for finding full-text information in print or electronic publications.

biological age: A reflection of TELOMERE attrition rate, meaning the rate at which the ends of the chromosome shorten. *See also* CHRONOLOGICAL AGE.

biomarkers: Physical indicators of a physiological or disease process; for example, high levels of CA125 in the blood may indicate ovarian cancer.

biotechnology: The application of engineering and technology principles to the life sciences.

blog: Web + log = blog. Typically, a blog is a personal journal that is published in the World Wide Web.

body mass index: An approximate measure of relative body fat that is calculated by dividing weight by height squared.

botanical: Relating to plants, or a medicine derived from plants.

browsers: *See* WEB BROWSERS.

carnitine: *See* ACETYL-L-CARNITINE.

carotenoids: Yellow or red PHYTOCHEMICALS thought to have health benefits. Examples include apricots, carrots, tomatoes, peaches, and corn.

cell death: Degeneration of cells in living organisms.

centenarians: Persons who are 100 years or older. *See also* NONAGENARIANS, OCTOGENARIANS.

channels: As related to Web sites, specific subsections of content. One site may have several channels devoted to specific topics or audiences.

chronological age: Actual age according to the calendar. *See also* BIOLOGICAL AGE.

clinical practice guidelines: Systematically developed directions for physicians and other health professionals to follow in specific medical circumstances.

clinical trials: Series of treatments used to evaluate the effectiveness of specific medications or medical procedures.

cognitive: Relating to mental processes including memory, reasoning, and comprehension.

consensus statements: An agreement on specific issues; related to medicine, these agreements form the basis of evidence-based practice, a framework for using the best scientific data to make decisions about the care and management of individual patients.

constituencies: Groups or categories of individuals, particularly in a specific geographic region.

correlation: The degree of association between two variables.

cryogenics: The study of the physiological effects of low temperatures. *Compare with* CRYONICS.

cryonics: The freezing and storage of human tissue, particularly from a dead body, for future use and/or rejuvenation. *Compare with* CRYOGENICS.

cytokines: PROTEINS that act as messengers that find and kill cancer cells, bacteria, and infected cells.

degenerative or **degeneration:** Deteriorating or showing loss of function.

dehydroepiandrosterone: DHEA, a hormone produced by the adrenal glands.

dementia: Deterioration of intellectual abilities such as memory, concentration, and judgment, due to a disease or a disorder of the brain.

demographics: Characteristics of a human population including age, gender, educational background, socioeconomic status, etc. *See also* DEMOGRAPHY.

demography: The study of populations including size, growth (birth and death rates), distribution, and density. *See also* DEMOGRAPHICS.

DHEA: Dehydroepiandrosterone, a hormone produced by the adrenal glands.

diagnosis: Methods used to identify characteristics, signs, or symptoms of a disease, condition, or ailment that distinguishes the disease from other diseases.

disease outbreaks: Sudden increases or eruptions of disease activity.

DNA: Deoxyribonucleic acid, the material inside cells that controls cell functions and controls the inheritance of traits and characteristics.

embryonic stem cells: *See* STEM CELLS.

epidemiology: The study of disease INCIDENCE, disease patterns, and DISEASE OUTBREAKS.

erectile dysfunction: Inability to maintain an erection and to ejaculate.

estrogen: A female sex HORMONE that is produced by the ovaries.

evidence-based medicine: The use of clinically relevant, published research to treat an individual patient. *See also* CONSENSUS STATEMENTS.

familial: Occurring in members of the same family.

fibroblasts: Cells present in connective tissue such as tendons and cartilage.

flavonoids: PHYTOCHEMICALS that are thought to have health benefits. Examples include the ANTHOCYANINS.

free radicals: *See* OXYGEN FREE RADICALS.

genetic: Relating to the science of GENETICS, or the mechanisms by which an organism's traits are inherited.

genetic engineering: The alteration of GENETIC MATERIAL in a living organism.

genetic material: This is a general term that covers organic human materials such as hair, saliva, and blood, as well as DNA sequences that have been extracted from human cells.

genetic mutation: Alteration or change of GENETIC MATERIAL.

genetically modified organisms: Plants or animals that have had their genetic makeup altered or modified in ways that could not be accomplished through normal reproduction. Foods that have been genetically modified are sometimes called NOVEL FOODS.

genetics: *See* GENETIC.

genome: An organism's GENETIC MATERIAL.

genomics: Study of the structure and function of GENETIC MATERIAL.

genotype: Genetic blueprint of an ORGANISM. *Compare with* PHENOTYPE.

geriatrics: The medical specialty that treats conditions and diseases related to old age. *Compare with* GERONTOLOGY.

gerontology: The scientific study of aging and old age. *Compare with* GERIATRICS.

glucose: A type of sugar that serves as the body's source of energy.

glycemic: Characteristic of having GLUCOSE in the blood.

gray literature: Publications that are not widely available through normal channels.

growth factors: PROTEINS that promote cell growth.

hormones: Substances that affect growth or METABOLISM.

hyperplasia: An abnormal increase in the amount of cells in tissues or an organ.

immune response: A physical response to an ANTIGEN by specific ANTIBODIES.

immunity: The ability to resist a specific desease due to previous exposure, immunization, or vaccination.

immunization: A procedure that introduces specific ANTIGENS to induce an IMMUNE RESPONSE, in an effort to improve the ability to resist infection, and to render IMMUNITY for a specific disease. This term is used interchangeably with VACCINATION.

immunoassays: Tests used to detect the presence or amount of substances that act as ANTIGENS or ANTIBODIES. *See also* ASSAYS.

impotence: Inability to maintain an erection and to ejaculate.

incidence: The rate of new cases of diseases or conditions in a specific population.

incontinence: Inability to control the elimination of feces and/or urine.

indolence: Laziness or inactivity.

inflammation: Response of body tissues to injury, infection, or foreign bodies including redness, swelling, and pain.

insomnia: Difficulty sleeping or a prolonged inability to sleep.

invisible Web: A term that refers to Internet content not easily accessible by normal search engines because of the way the information is organized.

L-carnitine: *See* ACETYL-L-CARNITINE.

lewy bodies: Round deposits in nerve cells, which can be significant in the diagnosis of a type of DEMENTIA.

libido: Sexual urge.

life expectancy: The number of years a person or group of persons is expected to live, based on statistical PROBABILITY. *See also* LIFE SPAN.

life span: Maximum age or length of life. *See also* LIFE EXPECTANCY.

lipoproteins: PROTEINS that carry fats in the blood.

longevity: The LIFE SPAN or length of life of an organism.

longitudinal studies: Studies that follow research subjects over a period of time.

lycopene: Red pigments in tomatoes, papayas, watermelons, and other ripe fruits that are believed to have health benefits.

macrobiotics: Dietary practice that features whole grains, cereals, beans, and vegetables.

macular: Relating to a part of the eye's RETINA.

maculopathy: Any disease of the macula lutea part of the eye.

MEDLINE: A bibliographic database of the published biomedical literature, developed by the U.S. National Library of Medicine (NLM). *See also* MEDLINEPLUS.

MedlinePlus: A consumer health resource developed by the National Library of Medicine that provides extensive information about more than 650 diseases and conditions. Also includes lists of hospitals and physicians, medical encyclopedia, medical dictionary, information about prescription and nonprescription drugs, and health information from the media. *See also* MEDLINE.

melanin: Skin pigment.

melatonin: A hormone that regulates brain activity.

meme: A behavioral value that is passed from one generation to another by means of imitation.

menopause: Change of life when menstrual periods cease, and the ovaries stop producing ESTROGEN.

metabolism: Chemical processes within a living organism.

metafilter: A type of BLOG that features content developed and posted by several persons.

micronutrients: Essential, nutritional elements that are needed in very small quantities. *See also* NUTRIENTS.

monographs: Books or detailed reports.

morbidity: Relative INCIDENCE or rate of disease.

mortality: Relative INCIDENCE or rate of death.

nanotechnology: Materials and processes that operate on the atomic and/or molecular level.

naturopathic medicine: Natural methods and therapies including nutrition, herbal medicines, and musculoskeletal manipulation. *See also* ALLOPATHIC MEDICINE.

nonagenarians: Persons aged ninety to ninety-nine years. *See also* CENTENARIANS, OCTOGENARIANS.

novel foods: GENETICALLY MODIFIED foods or foods that are new to a geographical region.

nutraceuticals: Foods or food supplements thought to have beneficial health effects.

nutrients: Substances such as trace elements that promote growth. *See also* MICRONUTRIENTS.

occurrence: Instances of a specific disease appearing in a population. *Compare with* INCIDENCE.

octogenarians: Persons aged eighty to eighty-nine years of age. *See also* CENTENARIANS, NONAGENARIANS.

ocular: Pertaining to the eye or vision.

organic: Related to or derived from living organisms.

organism: A living thing that functions independently.

outbreaks: *See* DISEASE OUTBREAKS.

oxidants: Substances that combine with oxygen and can cause disease. *See also* ANTIOXIDANTS, OXYGEN FREE RADICALS.

oxidative stress: A harmful state in which there are too many OXIDANTS, not enough antioxidants, and cell damage results.

oxygen free radicals: Oxygen molecules that remove electrons from molecules in healthy cells, thereby causing tissue and organ damage.

pathophysiology: Changes in physical functioning due to disease.

peer review: Professional evaluation of a colleague's work. This term usually refers to the evaluation of articles for publication or grants for funding.

pharmacopoeia: Compendium of drugs, chemicals, and other medicinal substances.

phenotype: Genetic traits that affect the actual appearance or behavior of an organism. Compare with GENOTYPE.

physiological age: An age that is consistent with the functioning of the body, which may be higher or lower than the CHRONOLOGICAL AGE. *See also* BIOLOGICAL AGE.

phytochemicals: Plant substances such as FLAVONOIDS or CAROTENOIDS which are thought to have health benefits.

placebo: An inactive substance that is used to test the effectiveness of another drug by comparing the results of the group that received the inactive substance and the group that received the active substance.

portals: As related to Web sites, gateways to resources.

practice guidelines: *See* CLINICAL PRACTICE GUIDELINES.

precocious: Exhibiting extremely early maturity.

presbycusis: Age-related hearing loss.

presbyopia: Age-related farsightedness.

primers: Introductory textbooks or guides.

probability: A measurement of the likelihood that an event will occur.

progeria: A disease that is characterized by the rapid onset of aging in childhood.

prognosis: Forecast or likely outcome of a disease or health condition.

prolapse: A slip or fall out of place, particularly an organ or anatomical structure such as the uterus or rectum.

proteinaceous: Related to protein or PROTEINS.

proteins: Complex ORGANIC substances essential for growth and repair of tissues in humans and animals. Proteins are commonly found in meat, eggs, dairy products, and some plant foods.

protocols: Related to the Internet, they are standards that govern communication and the transfer of data; related to science, they are standard procedures that govern scientific research studies.

quackery: Medicine practiced by a dishonest or unqualified individual. The term *quack* refers to unschooled, unskilled, or unscrupulous medical practitioners.

randomized controlled trials: Scientific studies that compare the results of one group that receives treatment or intervention and another group that receives no treatment or intervention. Randomized means that the researchers involved in the study assign patients randomly to the groups that will be compared.

rejuvenation: Restoration of youthfulness and vitality.

reliability: The degree to which a repeated measurement yields consistent results.

residue: In this context, the amount of a toxic substance that remains on surfaces, in the soil, or in plant or animal tissues.

retina: The part of the eye that receives and transmits optical images to the brain.

retinopathy: A disorder of the eye's RETINA that can lead to blindness.

retrospective studies: Reviews of previous cases or records in efforts to see patterns or common outcome.

risk/benefit ratios: Comparisons of relative health risks to relative health benefits.

RNA: Ribonucleic acid is a chemical found in the nucleus and cytoplasm of cells that carries GENETIC information to other parts of the cell where it is converted to proteins. *Compare with* DNA.

search directories: Web tools that organize Internet resources by subject and/or file type such as documents, images, or news group messages.

search engines: Web tools that find Internet resources based on key words or phrases typed into search interfaces.

secretion: Formation and release of body substances such as mucous or saliva.

secretogogues: Substances that stimulate SECRETION. For example, growth hormone or insulin.

senescence: The process of growing old, or the loss of function that can be attributed to the aging process.

senility: The state of being physically or mentally weak or ill due to age.

significance: Related to statistics, a measure that indicates whether an event or outcome is due to chance alone. An experiment is considered statistically significant if there is a less than one in twenty chance PROBABILITY that an event or outcome would have occurred anyway, regardless of intervention.

skepticism: A doubting or questioning outlook. A *skeptic* is a person who doubts or questions.

stem cells: Immature cells from which all blood cells are derived. Embryonic, fetal, adult, hematopoietic, and neural stem cells are being used in a variety of research experiments.

subsets: Parts of a larger collection.

sustainability: Practices used to maintain a healthy environment, particularly recycling.

synonyms: Words with similar meanings.

telomerase: An enzyme that maintains a chromosome's normal length. *See also* TELOMERES.

telomeres: Ends or tips of chromosomes where GENETIC information is located, and that shorten as cells age. Telomere attrition rate is a measure of BIOLOGICAL AGE. *See also* BIOMARKERS, TELOMERASE.

testosterone: A male sex hormone that is produced by the male reproductive organs.

think tanks: Organizations that study, research, and report on significant societal issues.

tissues: As related to the body, a collection of similar cells that act together and perform specific functions.

transhumanism: A philosophy that embraces life extension, CRYONICS, NANOTECHNOLOGY, and other techniques that strive to improve and/or extend life.

vaccination: See IMMUNIZATION.

validity: The extent to which a test measures what it is supposed to measure. *Compare with* RELIABILITY.

vegan: A person who eats only plant foods and no products that are derived from animals.

Web browsers: Software programs such as Netscape, Internet Explorer, or Firefox that are used to view content (text, images) on the World Wide Web.

Webcasts: Audio and/or video files that are broadcast on the World Wide Web in real time.

white papers: AUTHORITATIVE reports or position papers on issues of concern or controversy.

Bibliography

Anttila, T., Helkala, E.-L., Viitanen, M., Kareholt, I., Fratiglioni, L., Winblad, B., Soininen, H., Tuomilehto, J., Nissinen, A., and Kivipelto, M. (2004). "Alcohol Drinking in Middle Age and Subsequent Risk of Mild Cognitive Impairment and Dementia in Old Age: A Prospective Population Based Study." *BMJ* 329(August 10). DOI:10.1136/bmj.38181.418958.BE.

Baun, M. M., Oetting, K., and Bergstrom, N. (1991). "Health Benefits of Companion Animals in Relation to the Physiologic Indices of Relaxation." *Holistic Nursing Practice* 5(2): 16-23.

Gonos, Efstathios S. (2000). "Genetics of Aging: Lessons from Centenarians." *Experimental Gerontology* 35(February): 15-21.

Holmes, D. J. and Ottinger, M. A. (2003). "Birds As Long-Lived Animal Models for the Study of Aging." *Experimental Gerontology* 38(November-December): 1365-1375.

Louet, Sabine (2003). "Centenarians Provide Genetic Clue to Age-Related Disease." *Drug Discovery Today* 8(April): 280-281.

Sable, P. (1995). "Pets, Attachment, and Well-Being Across the Life Cycle." *Social Work* 40(3): 334-341.

Serpell, J. A. (1991) "Beneficial Effects of Pet Ownership on Some Aspects of Human Health and Behavior." *Journal of the Royal Society of Medicine* 84: 717-720.

Tse, Mimi M. Y. and Benzie, Iris F. F. (2004). "Diet and Health: Nursing Perspective for the Health of Our Aging Population." *Nursing & Health Sciences* 6(December): 309-314.

Index

Page numbers followed by the letter "f" indicate figures; those followed by the letter "t" indicate tables.

Exercise, health effects of, 26, 29, 60, 63, 64, 70, 95
Eye disorders, 43, 44, 51-52, 90, 94

Fasting, 29. *See also* Calorie restriction
Fecal incontinence, 45
Fennel, 78
Fiber, dietary, 57
Fibroblast growth factors, 79
File transfer protocol (FTP), 2
Fingernails, 42
Fish
    cold water, health effects of, 57, 61, 62
    oils, 61, 97
Fitness regimens. *See* Exercise, health effects of
Flavonoids, 55-59
Floaters (eye disorder), 52, 90
Food
    labels, 33
    macrobiotic, 61
    pigments, 58
    pyramid, 57, 61, 62f
    raw, 59-60, 62
    serving sizes, 17, 90
Forecasting, 101
Forgetfulness, 46-47
Frailty, 42, 77
Fraud, health, 10
Fries, James F., 78
Future forecasts, 101

Gait, 39
Gavrilov, Leonid A., 34-35, 105
Gavrilova, Natalia S., 34-35, 105
Genes
    cancer, 64
    longevity, 55, 86, 106
    testing, 64
    therapy, 31, 76-77
    tumor suppressor, 29
Genetic diseases, 26, 88, 92
Glaucoma, 51-52, 90

Glucose, 80
Glycemic index, 57, 60-61, 62
Gopher search tool, 5
Gotu kola, 78
Grabowski, Thomas J., 46
Growth
    factors, 52, 79
    hormones, 80-81

Hair disorders, 42, 43-44
Health
    on the Net (HON) Foundation, 4, 4f
    screening, 42, 52
Hearing loss, 26, 43, 44-45
Heart diseases, 24, 54, 58, 97
Hemoglobin disorders, 76
Herbs, 32, 55-56, 58, 77-79
Hip replacement, 40
HIV/AIDS, 21, 64
Hoaxes, 10
Hope, Bob, 85
Hormones
    DHEA, 30, 76, 79, 98
    growth. *See* Human growth hormones
    replacement therapy, 31, 48, 79, 80-81, 82
    testing, 30, 80
Human growth hormones, 30, 76, 79, 80, 81, 98
Hunger, 105
Hutchinson-Gilford Progeria syndrome, 85
Hypertension, 80

Immunizations in adults, 23, 32
Impotence. *See* Erectile dysfunction
Incontinence, 45-46, 49
Insomnia, 72-73
Intercourse, painful, 69
Invisible Web, 8-9

Japanese centenarians, 87
Java scripting, 3

For Product Safety Concerns and Information please contact our EU
representative GPSR@taylorandfrancis.com
Taylor & Francis Verlag GmbH, Kaufingerstraße 24, 80331 München, Germany